Alkaline Diet Cookbook

*Simple, balanced
and flavorful recipes
for a healthy lifestyle
or for an easy weight loss*

Isaac Vinson

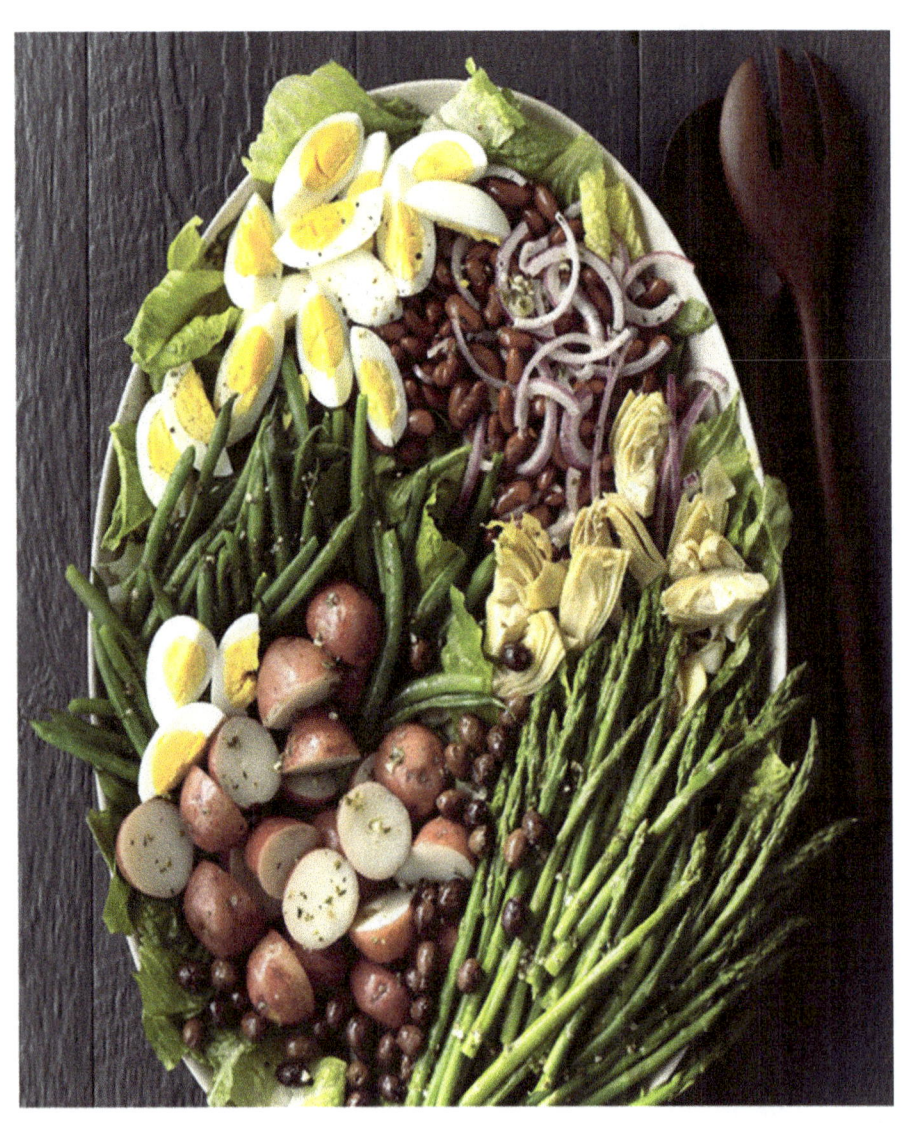

© **copyright 2021 – all rights reserved.**

the content contained within this book may not be reproduced, duplicated or transmitted without direct written permission from the author or the publisher.

under no circumstances will any blame or legal responsibility be held against the publisher, or author, for any damages, reparation, or monetary loss due to the information contained within this book. either directly or indirectly.

legal notice:

this book is copyright protected. this book is only for personal use. you cannot amend, distribute, sell, use, quote or paraphrase any part, or the content within this book, without the consent of the author or publisher.

disclaimer notice:

please note the information contained within this document is for educational and entertainment purposes only. all effort has been executed to present accurate, up to date, and reliable, complete information. no warranties of any kind are declared or implied. readers acknowledge that the author is not engaging in the rendering of legal, financial, medical or professional advice. the content within this book has been derived from various sources. please consult a licensed professional before attempting any techniques outlined in this book.

by reading this document, the reader agrees that under no circumstances is the author responsible for any losses, direct or indirect, which are incurred as a result of the use of information contained within this document, including, but not limited to, — errors, omissions, or inaccuracies.

Table of Contents

- Sweet and Sour Onions 5
- Sautéed Apples and Onions 7
- Zucchini Noodles with Portabella Mushrooms 9
- Grilled Tempeh with Pineapple 11
- Lentil-Stuffed Potato Cakes 13
- Sesame Ginger Cauliflower Rice 15
- Nori Wraps with Fresh Vegetables and Quinoa 17
- Kale Wraps with Chili, Garlic, and Green Beans 19
- Cabbage Wraps with Avocado, Asparagus, Pecan Nuts and Strawberries 22
- Millet Tabbouleh, Lime and Cilantro 24
- Lemony Salmon Burgers 26
- Caprese Turkey Burgers 28
- Pasta Salad 30
- Lemon-Thyme Eggs 32
- Spinach Salad with Bacon 34
- Pea and Collards Soup 36
- Spanish Stew 38
- Creamy Taco Soup 40
- Chicken with Caprese Salsa 43
- Balsamic-Roasted Broccoli 45
- Hearty Beef and Vegetable Soup 47
- Cauliflower Muffin 49
- Ham and Egg Cups 51
- Cauliflower Rice With Chicken 53
- Turkey With Fried Eggs 55
- Sweet Potato, Kale, and White Bean Stew 57
- Lighter Eggplant Parmesan 60
- Coconut-Lentil Curry 62
- Stuffed Portobello With Cheese 64
- Lighter Shrimp Scampi 67

Maple-Mustard Salmon	69
Chicken Salad With Grapes And Pecans	72
Courgettes In Cider Sauce	74
Baked Mixed Mushrooms	76
Spiced Okra	80
Alkalizing Green Soup	82
Healing Ginger Carrot Soup	84
Kale Salad	85
Turmeric Curry And Roasted Cauliflower	88
Alkaline Tortilla Soup	92
Hearty Minestrone	95
Raw Pad Thai (With Zucchini Noodles)	98
Spinach Quinoa	100
Spicy Eggplant	103

Sweet and Sour Onions

Preparation Time: 10 minutes
Cooking Time: 11 minutes
Servings: 4

Ingredients :

- 4 large onions, halved

- 2 garlic cloves, crushed

- 3 cups vegetable stock

- 1 ½ tablespoon balsamic vinegar

- ½ teaspoon Dijon mustard

- 1 tablespoon sugar

Directions:
1. Combine onions and garlic in a pan. Fry for 3 minutes, or till softened.

2. Pour stock, vinegar, Dijon mustard, and sugar. Bring to a boil.

3. Reduce heat. Cover and let the combination simmer for 10 minutes.

4. Get rid of from heat. Continue stirring until the liquid is reduced and the onions are brown. Serve.

Nutrition:
Calories 203

Total Fat 41. 2 g

Saturated Fat 0.8 g

Cholesterol 0 mg

Sodium 861 mg

Total Carbs 29. 5 g

Fiber 16. 3 g

Sugar 29. 3 g

Protein 19. 2 g

Sautéed Apples and Onions

Preparation Time: 14 minutes
Cooking Time: 16 minutes
Servings: 3

Ingredients :
- 2 cups dry cider

- 1 large onion, halved

- 2 cups vegetable stock

- 4 apples, sliced into wedges

- Pinch of salt

- Pinch of pepper

Directions:
1. Combine cider and onion in a saucepan. Bring to a boil until the onions are cooked and liquid almost gone.

2. Pour the stock and the apples. Season with salt and pepper. Stir occasionally. Cook for about 10 minutes or until the apples are tender but not mushy. Serve.

Nutrition:
Calories 343

Total Fat 51. 2 g

Saturated Fat 0.8 g

Cholesterol 0 mg

Sodium 861 mg

Total Carbs 22. 5 g

Fiber 6. 3 g

Sugar 2. 3 g

Protein 9. 2 g

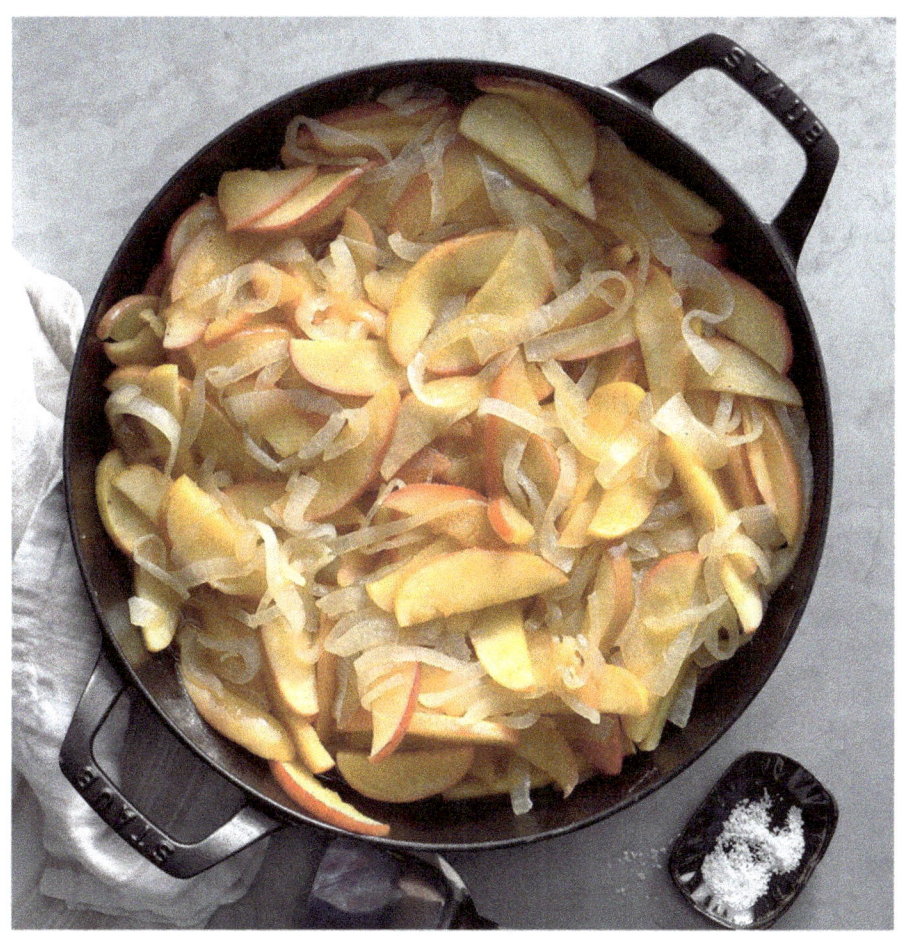

Zucchini Noodles with Portabella Mushrooms

Preparation Time: 14 minutes
Cooking Time: 16 minutes
Servings: 3

Ingredients :
- 1 zucchini, processed into spaghetti-like noodles
- 3 garlic cloves, minced
- 2 white onions, thinly sliced
- 1 thumb-sized ginger, julienned
- 1 lb. chicken thighs
- 1 lb. portabella mushrooms, sliced into thick slivers
- 2 cups chicken stock
- 3 cups water
- Pinch of sea salt, add more if needed
- Pinch of black pepper, add more if needed
- 2 tsp. sesame oil
- 4 Tbsp. coconut oil, divided
- ¼ cup fresh chives, minced, for garnish

Directions:
1. Pour 2 tablespoons of coconut oil into a large saucepan. Fry mushroom slivers in batches for 5 minutes or until seared brown. Set aside. Transfer these to a plate.

2. Sauté the onion, garlic, and ginger for 3 minutes or until tender. Add in chicken thighs, cooked mushrooms, chicken stock, water, salt, and pepper stir mixture well. Bring to a boil.

3. Decrease gradually the heat and allow simmering for 20 minutes or until the chicken is forking tender. Tip in sesame oil.

4. Serve by placing an equal amount of zucchini noodles into bowls. Ladle soup and garnish with chives.

Nutrition:
Calories 163

Total Fat 4. 2 g

Saturated Fat 0.8 g

Cholesterol 0 mg

Sodium 861 mg

Total Carbs 22. 5 g

Fiber 6. 3 g

Sugar 2. 3 g

Protein 9. 2 g

Grilled Tempeh with Pineapple

Preparation Time: 12 minutes
Cooking Time: 16 minutes
Servings: 3

Ingredients :
- 10 oz. tempeh, sliced

- 1 red bell pepper, quartered

- 1/4 pineapple, sliced into rings

- 6 oz. green beans

- 1 tbsp. coconut aminos

- 2 1/2 tbsp. orange juice, freshly squeeze

- 1 1/2 tbsp. lemon juice, freshly squeezed

- 1 tbsp. extra virgin olive oil

- 1/4 cup hoisin sauce

Directions:
1. Blend together the olive oil, orange and lemon juices, coconut aminos or soy sauce, and hoisin sauce in a bowl. Add the diced tempeh and set aside.

2. Heat up the grill or place a grill pan over medium high flame. Once hot, lift the marinated tempeh from the bowl with a pair of tongs and transfer them to the grill or pan.

3. Grille for 2 to 3 minutes, or until browned all over.

4. Grill the sliced pineapples alongside the tempeh, then transfer them directly onto the serving platter.

5. Place the grilled tempeh beside the grilled pineapple and cover with aluminium foil to keep warm.

6. Meanwhile, place the green beans and bell peppers in a bowl and add just enough of the marinade to coat.

7. Prepare the grill pan and add the vegetables. Grill until fork tender and slightly charred.

8. Transfer the grilled vegetables to the serving platter and arrange artfully with the tempeh and pineapple. Serve at once.

Nutrition:
Calories 163

Total Fat 4. 2 g

Saturated Fat 0.8 g

Cholesterol 0 mg

Sodium 861 mg

Total Carbs 22. 5 g

Fiber 6. 3 g

Sugar 2. 3 g

Protein 9. 2 g

Lentil-Stuffed Potato Cakes

Preparation Time: 15 Minutes
Cooking Time: 30 minutes
Servings: 4

Ingredients
- For the Cakes:

- Salt

- 1 bay leaf

- 10 medium gold potatoes

- 1 cup potato starch- add more for dusting

- For the Stuffing:

- Coconut oil for panfrying

- Salt and freshly ground black pepper

- 1 medium onion, chopped

- 4-ounces mushrooms

- 2 tablespoons olive oil

- ¾ cup dried green lentils (preferably French lentils)- cooked

Directions:
1. Combine the 7 cups of water, potatoes and bay leaf in a large pot and boil until the potatoes are tender. Poke with a fork to ensure they are cooked.

2. Rinse the potatoes under cold water when done; the skins will peel off easily. Now mash the potatoes until smooth and add the potato starch, stir to make dough. Add more potato starch if the dough feels too sticky.

3. For the stuffing, add olive oil to a sauté pan and place over medium high heat. Add in onions and cook as you stir for 5 minutes. Add in the lentils together with pepper and salt (to taste) and cook for 2 minutes. Set aside.

4. To make the cakes, scoop about 3 tablespoons of the dough on your hand and press it into your palm. Add a spoonful of stuffing on top of the dough and fold it over to close it. Shape it into a round disk.

5. Now add coconut oil to a skillet and heat over medium heat. Cook the potato cakes on both sides until golden, roughly 4 minutes per side.

Nutrition:
Calories: 197

Sesame Ginger Cauliflower Rice

Preparation Time: 10 Minutes
Cooking Time: 15 minutes
Servings: 4

Ingredients
- 2 tablespoons wheat-free tamari plus more to taste
- 4 cups finely chopped mushrooms
- 1 large head cauliflower
- 2 tablespoons toasted sesame oil
- 2 tablespoons grapeseed oil
- 1/2 teaspoon Celtic sea salt- plus more to taste
- 6 green onions- finely chopped (white and green parts)
- 1 bunch cilantro- finely chopped (1/2 cup)
- 2 tablespoons minced fresh ginger
- 2 teaspoons fresh lime juice- plus more to taste
- 1 small green chile- ribbed, seeded, and minced
- 4 teaspoons minced garlic (4 cloves)

Directions:
1. For the cauliflower rice, roughly cut the cauliflower into florets and get rid of the tough middle core.

2. Fit a food processor with an S blade and add the florets to pulse. Pulse for a few seconds until the florets achieve a rice like consistency. You should have 5 to 6 cups of rice in the end.

3. Heat oil in a deep skillet or wok over medium high heat and fry the ginger, green onions, chili, garlic and mushroom seasoned with ¼ teaspoon of salt for 5 minutes. Once combined well and soft, add in the tamari and cauliflower rice and cook for 5 more minutes until soft.

4. Add in remaining salt, cilantro, and lime juice and adjust the flavors as desired.

5. Serve and enjoy!

Nutrition:
Calories: 83

Nori Wraps with Fresh Vegetables and Quinoa

Preparation Time: 15 Minutes
Cooking Time: 20 minutes
Servings: 1

This is an extremely high nutrient alkaline diet for everyone out there. Quinoa, which is a source of protein, is considered the only 100% protein plant around. It is rich in fiber and other essential nutrients.

Nori (seaweed), on the other hand, is antioxidant and rich in nutrients.

When you put everything together, the Ingredients in this diet will leave your stomach satisfied, your body nourished and your taste bud happy, all at the same time.

Ingredients :
- Nori sheets, two (2)
- Raw carrot sticks, ¼ cup (60ml)
- Cooked quinoa, ½ cup (125 ml)
- Raw carrot sticks, ¼ cup (60ml)
- Fresh garlic, finely chopped, one (1) teaspoon (5ml)
- Raw seed mix, one (1) tablespoon (15ml)

- Fresh ginger root, finely grated, one (1) teaspoon (5ml)
- Raw cucumber sticks, ¼ cup (60ml)
- Fresh coriander leaves, finely chopped, ¼ cup (60ml)
- Sesame oilseed, one (1) tablespoon (15ml)

Directions:
1. Get a bowl and mix cooked quinoa with coriander leaves, ginger, seed mix, coriander leaves, and garlic.

2. Pour the sesame oil seed and mix properly.

3. Spread out both nori sheets on two surfaces.

4. Spread the quinoa mix one each nori sheets.

5. Add carrot sticks and cucumber on top of the quinoa.

6. Fold up the nori sheets with the quinoa Ingredients inside.

7. Depending on how you like it, serve with pickled ginger or soy sauce.

Nutrition:
Calories: 160

Kale Wraps with Chili, Garlic, and Green Beans

Preparation Time: 30 Minutes
Cooking Time: 0 minutes
Servings: 2

The **Ingredients** that make up this diet are incredibly nutritious to the body. Let's start with Green beans – they are rich in fiber and also serve as a cleansing agent to the colon.

Kale is extremely useful when it comes to detoxifying the body because it helps in cleansing the kidney.

The Avocado and raw seed mix are replete with cholesterol-lowering fat, which is essential in keeping the body healthy.

And Coriander, on the other hand, remains a real source for essential nutrients and fiber.

Now, when you consider everything put together, this meal is highly nutritious, healthy and delicious. The best part is, it's alkaline.

Ingredients :
1. Fresh lime juice (30ml), one (1) tablespoon

2. Raw seed mix (15ml), one (1) tablespoon

3. Kale leaves (large), two (2)

4. Fresh garlic (finely chopped, 10ml), two (2) teaspoons

5. Ripe avocado (pitted and sliced), half (½)

6. Fresh red chili (seeded & finely chopped), one (1) teaspoon (5ml)

7. Fresh cucumber sticks (250ml), one (10) cup

8. Fresh coriander leaves (finely chopped), (125ml), ½ cup

9. Green beans (250ml), one (1) cup

Directions:
1. Spread kale leaves on a clean kitchen work surface.

2. Spread each chopped coriander leaves on each leaf, position them around the end of the leaf, perpendicular to the edge.

3. Spread green beans equally on each leaf, at the edge of each leaf, same as the coriander leaves.

4. Do the same thing with the cucumber sticks.

5. Cut the divide chopped garlic across each leaf, sprinkling it all over the green beans.

6. Cut and share the chopped chili across each leaf and sprinkle it over the garlic.

7. Now, divide the avocado across each leaf, and spread it over chili, garlic, coriander and green beans.

8. Share the raw seed mix among each leaf, and sprinkle them over other Ingredients.

9. Divide the lime juice on across each leaf and drizzle it over all other Ingredients.

10. Now fold or roll up the kale leaves and wrap up all the Ingredients within it.

11. You can serve with soy sauce!

Nutrition:
Calories: 298

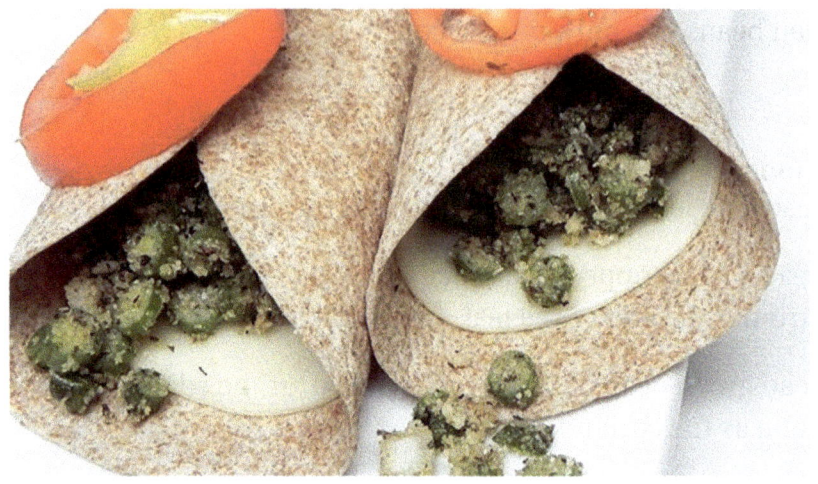

Cabbage Wraps with Avocado, Asparagus, Pecan Nuts and Strawberries

Preparation Time: 30 Minutes
Cooking Time: 0 minutes
Servings: 1

The Cabbage wraps with avocado, asparagus, pecan nuts, and strawberries is another delicious and powerful alkaline diet at your service.

If you are conscious of your health, there is every possibility that you must have heard about the alkaline diet and how it helps stabilize the human body pH. The Ingredients in this meal are super rich in nutrients, e.g., in as much as strawberries are natural sweeteners, they are also anti-oxidants. Asparagus, on the other hand, possess an inherent property that helps mitigate aging. Its ability to help drain the liver is also an impressive feature in the process of detoxification.

It is exceptionally delicious and healthy.

Ingredients :
- Raw pecan nuts (roughly chopped), 125 ml, ½ cup

- Fresh sliced strawberries, 124 ml, ½ cup

- Cabbage leaves, two (2) large

- Ripe avocado (pitted & sliced), ½
- Green asparagus spears (250 ml), one (1) cup

Directions:
1. Spread out the cabbage sheets on a clean kitchen work surface.

2. Share the asparagus shear among each cabbage leaf and place them on the edge of the leaf.

3. Share the avocado slices on each leaf and put them on top of the asparagus spears.

4. Share the strawberries over each leaf and spread on top of the avocado slices.

5. Share the pecan nuts between each leaf and spread it on the strawberries.

6. Wrap the leaves with all Ingredients inside them.

7. Serve with soy sauce (optional).

8. Enjoy.

Nutrition:
Calories: 146

Millet Tabbouleh, Lime and Cilantro

Preparation Time: 15 Minutes
Cooking Time: 20 minutes
Servings: 6

This super alkaline delicacy is tasty, nutritious, and filling. The Ingredients that make up this meal are millet, tomatoes, lime juice, hot sauce, olive oil, green onions, cucumber, and cilantro.

The Millet Tabbouleh, Lime, and Cilantro recipe is guaranteed to keep your blood pH alkaline, which in turn translates to healthy living, productiveness, and happiness.

Enjoy this recipe.

Ingredients :
- Lime juice, ½ cup

- Cilantro (chopped), ½ cup

- Hot sauce, 5-6 drops (Tabasco)

- Olive oil, ¼ cup and two (2) teaspoons (divided)

- Tomatoes (diced), two (2) large

- Green onions, two (2) bunches

- Cucumber (peeled, seeded and juiced), two (2)

- Millet (rinsed and drained), one (1) cup

Directions:
1. Heat olive oil in a saucepan over medium heat.

2. Add the millet and fry until it begins to smell fragrant (this takes between three (3) to four (4) minutes).

3. Add about six (6) cups of water and bring to boil.

4. Wait for about fifteen (15) minutes.

5. Turn off the heat, wash and rinse under cold water.

6. Drain the millet and transfer to a large bowl.

7. Add cucumbers, tomatoes, lime juice, cilantro, green onions, the ¼ cup oil, and hot sauce.

8. Season with pepper and salt to taste.

Nutrition:
Calories: 240

Lemony Salmon Burgers

Preparation Time: 10 Minutes
Cooking Time: 10 Minutes
Servings: 4

Ingredients
- 2 (3-oz) cans boneless, skinless pink salmon

- 1/4 cup panko breadcrumbs

- 4 tsp. lemon juice

- 1/4 cup red bell pepper

- 1/4 cup sugar-free yogurt

- 1 egg

- 2 (**1.** 5-oz) whole wheat hamburger toasted buns

Directions:
1. Mix drained and flaked salmon, finely-chopped bell pepper, panko breadcrumbs.

2. Combine 2 tbsp. cup sugar-free yogurt, 3 tsp. fresh lemon juice, and egg in a bowl. Shape mixture into 2 (3-inch) patties, bake on the skillet over medium heat 4 to 5 Minutes per side.

3. Stir together 2 tbsp. sugar-free yogurt and 1 tsp. lemon juice; spread over bottom halves of buns.

4. Top each with 1 patty, and cover with bun tops.

This dish is very mouth-watering!

Nutrition:
Calories 131

Protein 12

Fat 1 g

Carbs 19 g

Caprese Turkey Burgers

Preparation Time: 10 Minutes
Cooking Time: 10 Minutes
Servings: 4

Ingredients
- 1/2 lb. 93% lean ground turkey

- 2 (1,5-oz) whole wheat hamburger buns (toasted)

- 1/4 cup shredded mozzarella cheese (part-skim)

- 1 egg

- 1 big tomato

- 1 small clove garlic

- 4 large basil leaves

- 1/8 tsp. salt

- 1/8 tsp. pepper

Directions:
1. Combine turkey, white egg, Minced garlic, salt, and pepper (mix until combined);

2. Shape into 2 cutlets. Put cutlets into a skillet; cook 5 to 7 Minutes per side.

3. Top cutlets properly with cheese and sliced tomato at the end of cooking.

4. Put 1 cutlet on the bottom of each bun.

5. Top each patty with 2 basil leaves. Cover with bun tops.

My guests enjoy this dish every time they visit my home.

Nutrition:
Calories 180

Protein 7 g

Fat 4 g

Carbs 20 g

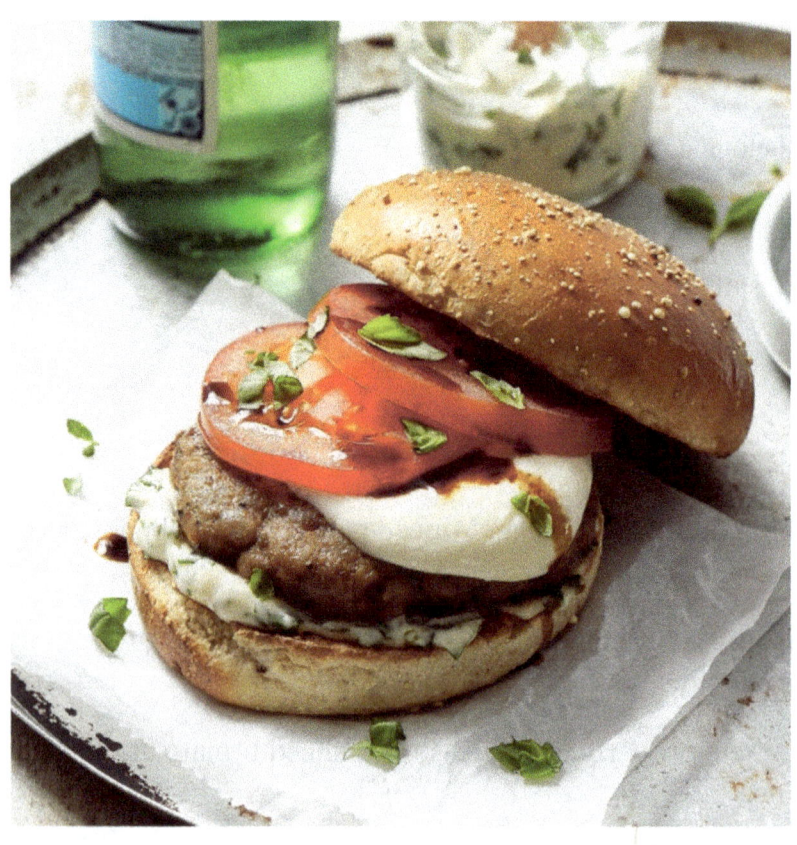

Pasta Salad

Preparation Time: 15 Minutes
Cooking Time: 15 Minutes
Servings: 4

Ingredients
- 8 oz. whole-wheat pasta
- 2 tomatoes
- 1 (5-oz) pkg spring mix
- 9 slices bacon
- 1/3 cup mayonnaise (reduced-fat)
- 1 tbsp. Dijon mustard
- 3 tbsp. apple cider vinegar
- 1/4 tsp. salt
- 1/2 tsp. pepper

Directions:
1. Cook pasta.

2. Chilled pasta, chopped tomatoes and spring mix in a bowl.

3. Crumble cooked bacon over pasta.

4. Combine mayonnaise, mustard, vinegar, salt and pepper in a small bowl.

5. Pour dressing over pasta, stirring to coat.

Understanding diabetes is the first step in curing.

Nutrition:
Calories 200

Protein 15 g

Fat 3 g

Carbs 6 g

Lemon-Thyme Eggs

Preparation Time: 10 Minutes
Cooking Time: 5 Minutes
Servings: 4

Ingredients
- 7 large eggs

- 1/4 cup mayonnaise (reduced-fat)

- 2 tsp. lemon juice

- 1 tsp. Dijon mustard

- 1 tsp. chopped fresh thyme

- 1/8 tsp. cayenne pepper

Directions:
1. Bring eggs to a boil.

2. Peel and cut each egg in half lengthwise.

3. Remove yolks to a bowl. Add mayonnaise, lemon juice, mustard, thyme, and cayenne to egg yolks; mash to blend. Fill egg white halves with yolk mixture.

4. Chill until ready to serve.

Please your family with a delicious meal.

Nutrition:
Calories 40

Protein 10 g

Fat 6 g

Carbs 2 g

Spinach Salad with Bacon

Preparation Time: 15 Minutes
Cooking Time: 0 Minutes
Servings: 4

Ingredients
- 8 slices center-cut bacon
- 3 tbsp. extra virgin olive oil
- 1 (5-oz) pkg baby spinach
- 1 tbsp. apple cider vinegar
- 1 tsp. Dijon mustard
- 1/2 tsp. honey
- 1/4 tsp. salt
- 1/2 tsp. pepper

Directions:
1. Mix vinegar, mustard, honey, salt and pepper in a bowl.

2. Whisk in oil. Place spinach in a serving bowl; drizzle with dressing, and toss to coat.

3. Sprinkle with cooked and crumbled bacon.

Nutrition:
Calories 110

Protein 6 g

Fat 2 g

Carbs 1 g

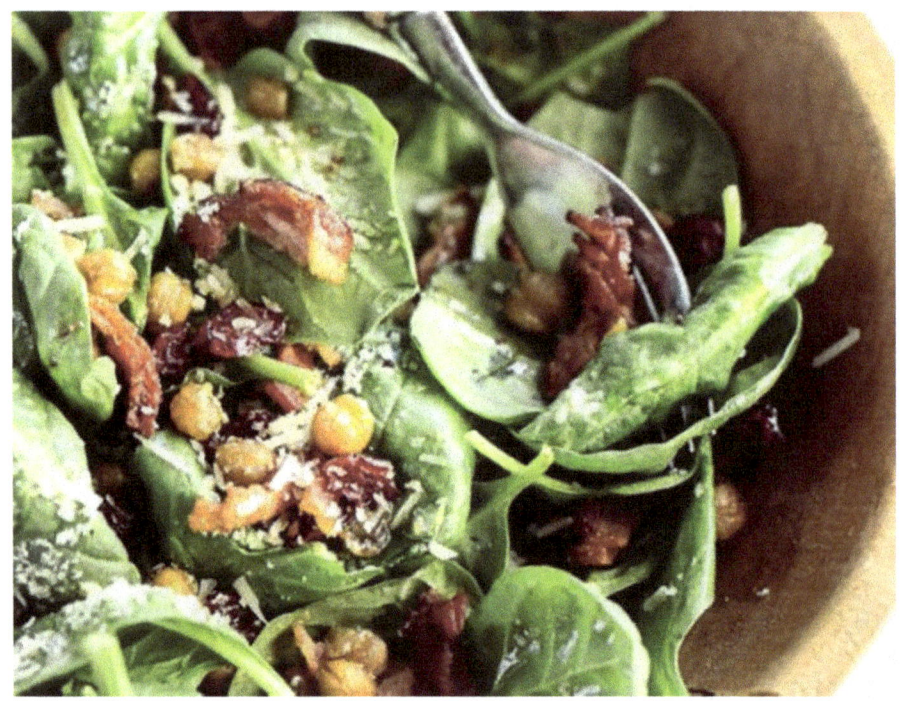

Pea and Collards Soup

Preparation Time: 10 Minutes
Cooking Time: 30 Minutes
Servings: 4

Ingredients
- 1/2 (16-oz) pkg black-eyed peas

- 1 onion

- 2 carrots

- 1,5 cups ham (low-sodium)

- 1 (1-lb) bunch collard greens (trimmed)

- 1 tbsp. extra virgin olive oil

- 2 cloves garlic

- 1/2 tsp. black pepper

- Hot sauce

Directions:
1. Cook chopped onion and carrots 10 Minutes.

2. Add peas, diced ham, collards, and Minced garlic. Cook 5 Minutes.

3. Add broth, 3 cups water, and pepper. Bring to a boil; simmer 35 Minutes, adding water if needed.

Serve with favorite sauce.

Nutrition:
Calories 86

Protein 15 g

Fat 2 g

Carbs 9 g

Spanish Stew

Preparation Time: 10 Minutes
Cooking Time: 25 Minutes
Servings: 4

Ingredients
- **1.** 1/2 (12-oz) pkg smoked chicken sausage links

- 1 (5-oz) pkg baby spinach

- 1 (15-oz) can chickpeas

- 1 (14. 5-oz) can tomatoes with basil, garlic, and oregano

- 1/2 tsp. smoked paprika

- 1/2 tsp. cumin

- 3/4 cup onions

- 1 tbsp. extra virgin olive oil

Directions:
1. Cook sliced the sausage in hot oil until browned. Remove from pot.

2. Add chopped onions; cook until tender.

3. Add sausage, drained and rinsed chickpeas, diced tomatoes, paprika, and ground cumin. Cook 15 Minutes.

4. Add in spinach; cook 1 to 2 Minutes.

This dish is ideal for every day and for a festive table.

Nutrition:
Calories 200

Protein 10 g

Fat 20 g

Carbs 1 g

Creamy Taco Soup

Preparation Time: 10 Minutes
Cooking Time: 20 Minutes
Servings: 4

Ingredients
- 3/4 lb. ground sirloin

- 1/2 (8-oz) cream cheese

- 1/2 onion

- 1 clove garlic

- 1 (10-oz) can tomatoes and green chiles

- 1 (14. 5-oz) can beef broth

- 1/4 cup heavy cream

- 1,5 tsp. cumin

- 1/2 tsp. chili powder

Directions:
1. Cook beef, chopped onion, and Minced garlic until meat is browned and crumbly; drain and return to pot.

2. Add ground cumin, chili powder, and cream cheese cut into small pieces and softened, stirring until cheese is melted.

3. Add diced tomatoes, broth, and cream; bring to a boil, and simmer 10 Minutes. Season with pepper and salt to taste.

You've got to give someone the recipe for this soup dish!

Nutrition:
Calories 60

Protein 3 g

Fat 1 g

Carbs 8 g

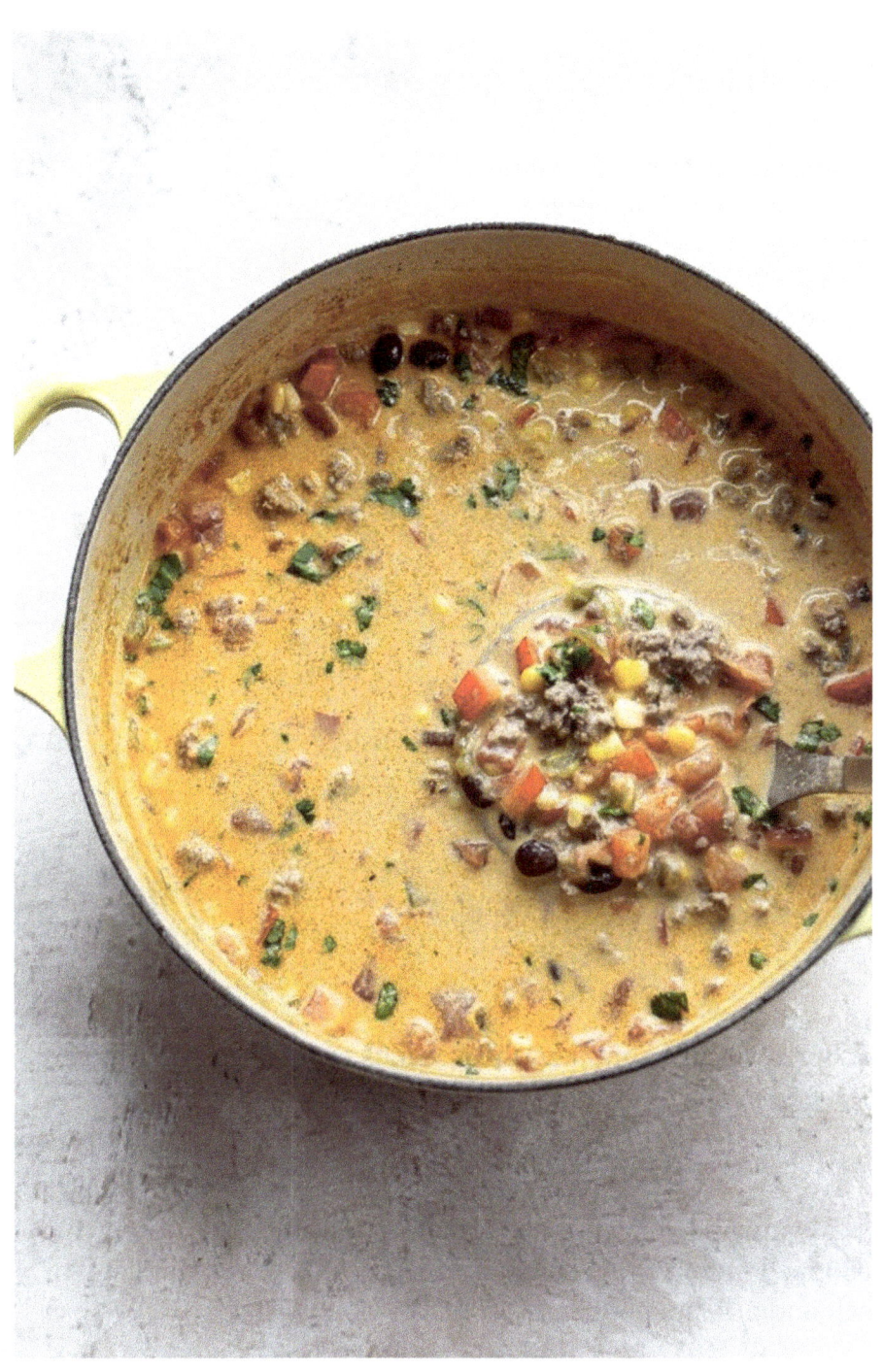

Chicken with Caprese Salsa

Preparation Time: 15 Minutes
Cooking Time: 5 Minutes
Servings: 4

Ingredients
- 3/4 lb. boneless, skinless chicken breasts

- 2 big tomatoes

- 1/2 (8-oz) ball fresh mozzarella cheese

- 1/4 cup red onion

- 2 tbsp. fresh basil

- 1 tbsp. balsamic vinegar

- 2 tbsp. extra virgin olive oil (divided)

- 1/2 tsp. salt (divided)

- 1/4 tsp. pepper (divided)

Directions:
1. Sprinkle cut in half lengthwise chicken with 1/4 tsp. salt and 1/8 tsp. pepper.

2. Heat 1 tbsp. olive oil, cook chicken 5 Minutes.

3. Meanwhile, mix chopped tomatoes, diced cheese, finely chopped onion, chopped basil, vinegar, 1 tbsp. oil, and 1/4 tsp. salt and 1/8 tsp. pepper.

4. Spoon salsa over chicken.

Chicken with Caprese Salsa is a nutritious, simple and very tasty dish that can be prepared in a few Minutes.

Nutrition:
Calories 210

Protein 28 g

Fat 17 g

Carbs 0, 1 g

Balsamic-Roasted Broccoli

Preparation Time: 10 Minutes
Cooking Time: 15 Minutes
Servings: 4

Ingredients
- 1 lb. broccoli

- 1 tbsp. extra virgin olive oil

- 1 tbsp. balsamic vinegar

- 1 clove garlic

- 1/8 tsp. salt

- Pepper to taste

Directions

1. Preheat oven to 450F.

2. Combine broccoli, olive oil, vinegar, Minced garlic, salt, and pepper; toss.

3. Spread broccoli on a baking sheet.

4. Bake 12 to 15 Minutes.

5. Really good!

Nutrition:
Calories 27

Protein 3 g

Fat 0, 3 g

Carbs 4 g

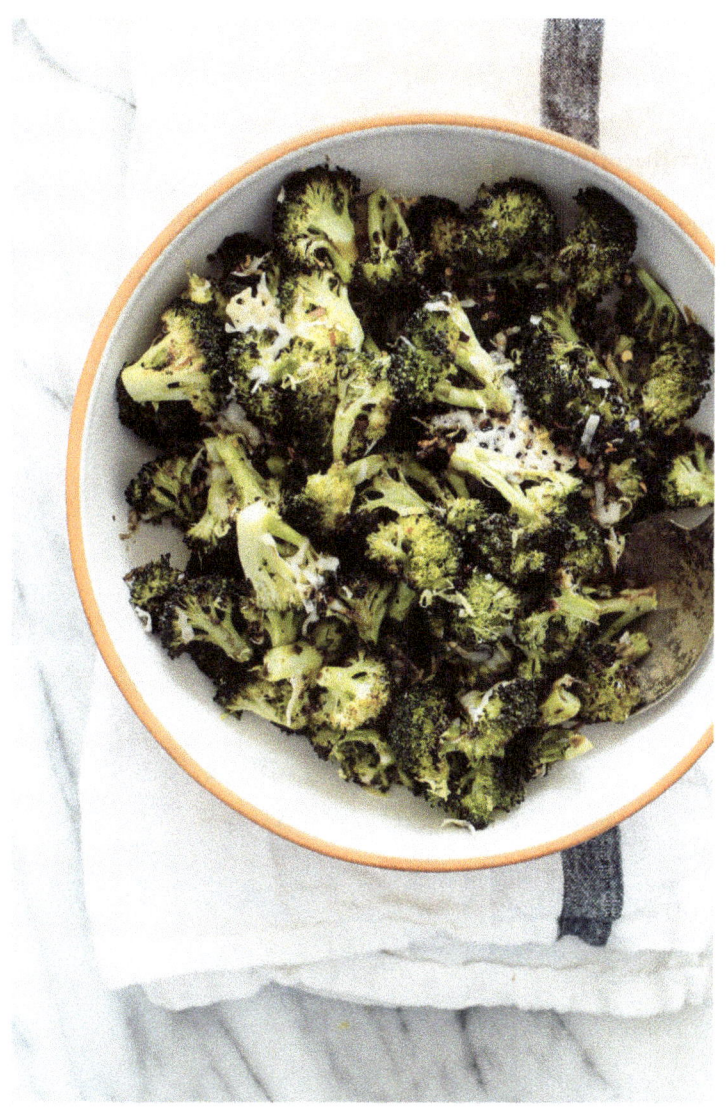

Hearty Beef And Vegetable Soup

Preparation Time: 10 Minutes
Cooking Time: 30 Minutes
Servings: 4

Ingredients
- 1/2 lb. lean ground beef

- 2 cups beef broth

- 1,5 tbsp. vegetable oil (divided)

- 1 cup green bell pepper

- 1/2 cup red onion

- 1 cup green cabbage

- 1 cup frozen mixed vegetables

- 1/2 can tomatoes

- 1,5 tsp. Worcestershire sauce

- 1 small bay leaf

- 1,8 tsp. pepper

- 2 tbsp. ketchup

Directions:
1. Cook beef in 1/2 tbsp. hot oil 2 Minutes.

2. Stir in chopped bell pepper and chopped onion; cook 4 Minutes.

3. Add chopped cabbage, mixed vegetables, stewed tomatoes, broth, Worcestershire sauce, bay leaf, and pepper; bring to a boil.

4. Reduce heat to medium; cover, and cook 15 Minutes.

5. Stir in ketchup and 1 tbsp. oil, and remove from heat. Let stand 10 Minutes.

The right diet is excellent diabetes remedy.

Nutrition:
Calories 170

Protein 17 g

Fat 8 g

Carbs 3 g

Cauliflower Muffin

Preparation Time: 15 Minutes
Cooking Time: 30 Minutes
Servings: 4

Ingredients
- 2,5 cup cauliflower

- **Servings:** cup ham
- 2,5 cups of cheese

- **Servings:** cup champignon

- 1,5 tbsp. flaxseed

- 3 eggs

- 1/4 tsp. salt

- 1/8 tsp. pepper

Directions:
1. Preheat oven to 375 F.

2. Put muffin liners in a 12-muffin tin.

3. Combine diced cauliflower, ground flaxseed, beaten eggs, cup diced ham, grated cheese, and diced mushrooms, salt, pepper.

4. Divide mixture rightly between muffin liners.

5. Bake 30 Minutes.

This is a great lunch for the whole family.

Nutrition:
Calories 116

Protein 10 g

Fat 7 g

Carbs 3 g

Ham And Egg Cups

Preparation Time: 10 Minutes
Cooking Time: 15 Minutes
Servings: 4

Ingredients
- 5 slices ham

- 4 tbsp. cheese

- 1,5 tbsp. cream

- 3 egg whites

- 1,5 tbsp. pepper (green)

- 1 tsp. salt

- pepper to taste

Directions:
1. Preheat oven to 350 F.

2. Arrange each slice of thinly sliced ham into 4 muffin tin.

3. Put 1/4 of grated cheese into ham cup.

4. Mix eggs, cream, salt and pepper and divide it into 2 tins.

5. Bake in oven 15 Minutes; after baking, sprinkle with green onions.

If you want to keep your current shape, also pay attention to this dish.

Nutrition:
Calories 180

Protein 13 g

Fat 13 g

Carbs 2 g

Cauliflower Rice With Chicken

Preparation Time: 15 Minutes
Cooking Time: 15 Minutes
Servings: 4

Ingredients
- 1/2 large cauliflower

- 3/4 cup cooked meat

- 1/2 bell pepper

- 1 carrot

- 2 ribs celery

- 1 tbsp. stir fry sauce (low carb)

- 1 tbsp. extra virgin olive oil

- Salt and pepper to taste

Directions:
1. Chop cauliflower in a processor to "rice." Place in a bowl.

2. Properly chop all vegetables in a food processor into thin slices.

3. Add cauliflower and other plants to WOK with heated oil. Fry until all veggies are tender.

4. Add chopped meat and sauce to the wok and fry 10 Minutes.

Serve.

This dish is very mouth-watering!

Nutrition:
Calories 200

Protein 10 g

Fat 12 g

Carbs 10 g

Turkey With Fried Eggs

Preparation Time: 10 Minutes
Cooking Time: 20 Minutes
Servings: 4

Ingredients
- 4 large potatoes

- 1 cooked turkey thigh

- 1 large onion (about 2 cups diced)

- butter

- Chile flakes

- 4 eggs

- salt to taste

- pepper to taste

Directions:
1. Rub the cold boiled potatoes on the coarsest holes of a box grater. Dice the turkey.

2. Cook the onion in as much unsalted butter as you feel comfortable with until it's just fragrant and translucent.

3. Add the rubbed potatoes and a cup of diced cooked turkey, salt and pepper to taste, and cook 20 Minutes.

Top each with a fried egg. Yummy!

Nutrition:
Calories 170

Protein 19 g

Fat 7 g

Carbs 6 g

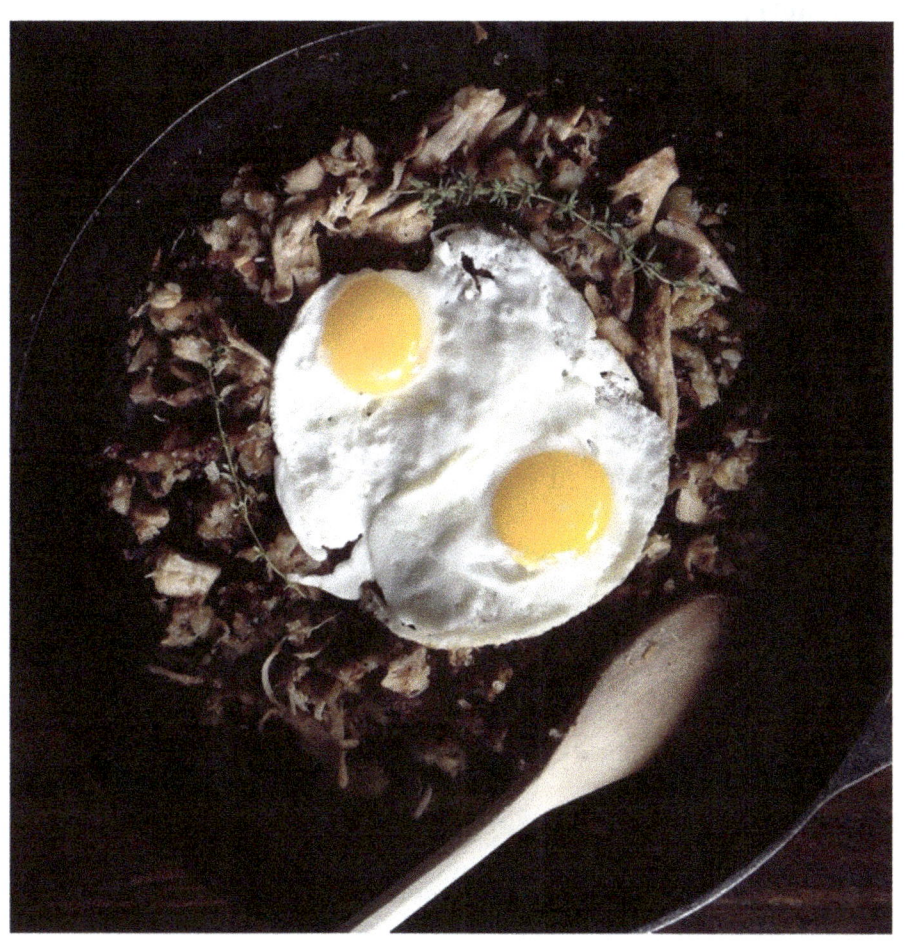

Sweet Potato, Kale, And White Bean Stew

Preparation Time: 15 minutes
Cooking Time: 25 minutes
Servings: 4

Ingredients :
- 1 (15-ounce) can low-sodium cannellini beans, rinsed and drained, divided

- 1 tablespoon olive oil

- 1 medium onion, chopped

- 2 garlic cloves, minced

- 2 celery stalks, chopped

- 3 medium carrots, chopped

- 2 cups low-sodium vegetable broth

- 1 teaspoon apple cider vinegar

- 2 medium sweet potatoes (about 1¼ pounds)

- 2 cups chopped kale

- 1 cup shelled edamame

- ¼ cup quinoa

- 1 teaspoon dried thyme

- 1/2 teaspoon cayenne pepper

- 1/2 teaspoon salt

- ¼ teaspoon freshly ground black pepper

Directions:
1. Put half the beans into a blender and blend until smooth. Set aside.

2. In a large soup pot over medium heat, heat the oil. When the oil is shining, include the onion and garlic, and cook until the onion softens and the garlic is sweet, about 3 minutes. Add the celery and carrots, and continue cooking until the vegetables soften, about 5 minutes.

3. Add the broth, vinegar, sweet potatoes, unblended beans, kale, edamame, and quinoa, and bring the mixture to a boil. Reduce the heat and simmer until the vegetables soften, about 10 minutes.

4. Add the blended beans, thyme, cayenne, salt, and black pepper, increase the heat to medium-high, and bring the mixture to a boil. Reduce the heat and simmer, uncovered, until the flavors combine, about 5 minutes.

5. Into each of 4 containers, scoop 1¾ cups of stew.

Nutrition:
calories: 373;

total fat: 7g;

saturated fat: 1g;

protein: 15g;

total carbs: 65g;

fiber: 15g;

sugar: 13g;

sodium: 540mg

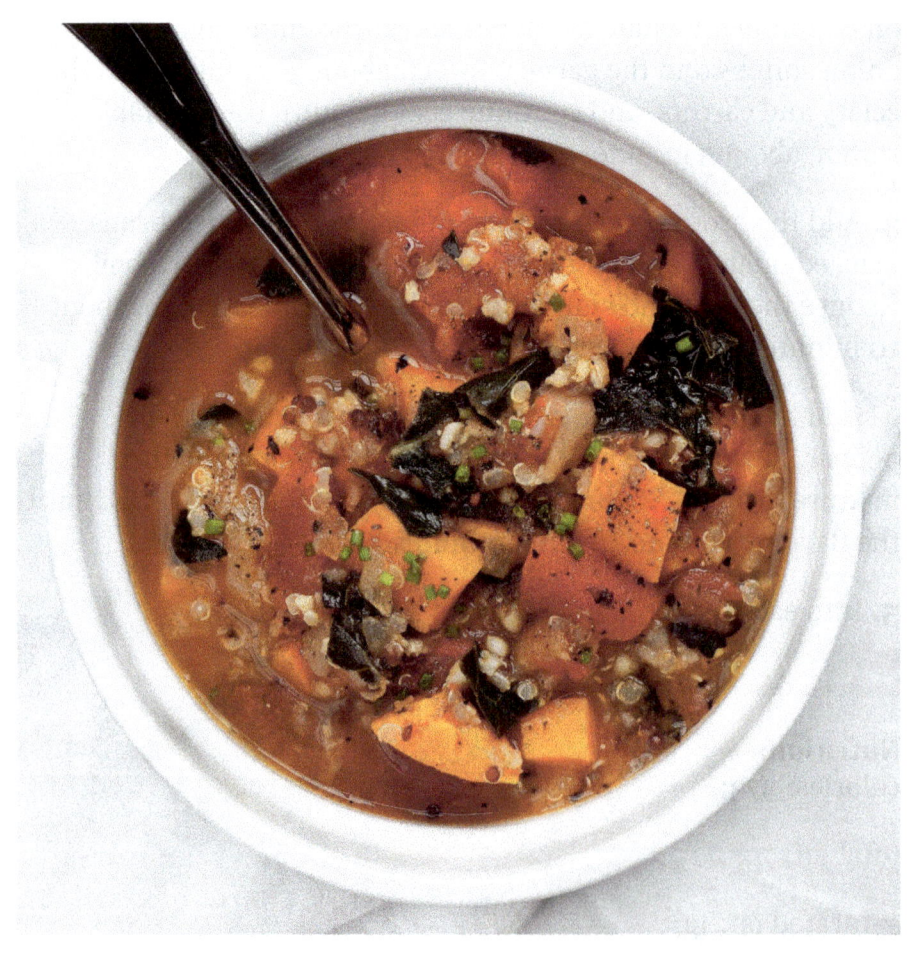

Lighter Eggplant Parmesan

Preparation Time: 15 minutes
Cooking Time: 35 minutes
Servings: 4

Ingredients :
- Nonstick cooking spray

- 3 eggs, beaten

- 1 tablespoon dried parsley

- 2 teaspoons ground oregano

- 1/8 teaspoon freshly ground black pepper

- 1 cup panko bread crumbs, preferably whole-wheat

- 1 large eggplant (about 2 pounds)

- 5 servings (21/2 cups) chunky tomato sauce or jarred low-sodium tomato sauce

- 1 cup part-skim mozzarella cheese

- ¼ cup grated parmesan cheese

Directions:
1. Preheat the oven to 450f. Coat a baking sheet with cooking spray.

2. In a medium bowl, whisk together the eggs, parsley, oregano, and pepper.

3. Pour the panko into a separate medium bowl.

4. Slice the eggplant into ¼-inch-thick slices. Dip each slice of eggplant into the egg mixture, shaking off the excess. Then dredge both sides of the eggplant in the panko bread crumbs. Place the coated eggplant on the prepared baking sheet, leaving a 1/2-inch space between each slice.

5. Bake for about 15 minutes until soft and golden brown. Remove from the oven and set aside to slightly cool.

6. Pour 1/2 cup of chunky tomato sauce on the bottom of an 8-by-15-inch baking dish. Using a spatula or the back of a spoon spread the tomato sauce evenly. Place half the slices of cooked eggplant, slightly overlapping, in the dish, and top with 1 cup of chunky tomato sauce, 1/2 cup of mozzarella and 2 tablespoons of grated parmesan. Repeat the layer, ending with the cheese.

7. Bake uncovered for 20 minutes until the cheese is bubbling and slightly browned.

8. Remove from the oven and allow cooling for 15 minutes before dividing the eggplant equally into 4 separate containers.

Nutrition:
calories: 333;

total fat: 14g;

saturated fat: 6g;

protein: 20g;

total carbs: 35g;

fiber: 11g;

sugar: 15g;

sodium: 994mg

Coconut-Lentil Curry

Preparation Time: 15 minutes
Cooking Time: 35 minutes
Servings: 4
Ingredients :
- 1 tablespoon olive oil

- 1 medium yellow onion, chopped

- 1 garlic clove, minced

- 1 medium red bell pepper, diced

- 1 (15-ounce) can green or brown lentils, rinsed and drained

- 2 medium sweet potatoes, washed, peeled, and cut into bite-size chunks (about 1¼ pounds)

- 1 (15-ounce) can no-salt-added diced tomatoes

- 2 tablespoons tomato paste

- 4 teaspoons curry powder

- 1/8 teaspoon ground cloves

- 1 (15-ounce) can light coconut milk

- ¼ teaspoon salt

- 2 pieces whole-wheat naan bread, halved, or 4 slices crusty bread

Directions:
1. In a large saucepan over medium heat, heat the olive oil. When the oil is shimmering, add both the onion and garlic and

cook until the onion softens and the garlic is sweet, for about 3 minutes.

2. Add the bell pepper and continue cooking until it softens, about 5 minutes more. Add the lentils, sweet potatoes, tomatoes, tomato paste, curry powder, and cloves, and bring the mixture to a boil. Reduce the heat to medium-low, cover, and simmer until the potatoes are softened, about 20 minutes.

3. Add the coconut milk and salt, and return to a boil. Reduce the heat and simmer until the flavors combine, about 5 minutes.

4. Into each of 4 containers, spoon 2 cups of curry.

5. Enjoy each serving with half of a piece of naan bread or 1 slice of crusty bread.

Nutrition:
calories: 559;

total fat: 16g;

saturated fat: 7g;

protein: 16g;

total carbs: 86g;

fiber: 16g;

sugar: 18g;

sodium: 819mg

Stuffed Portobello With Cheese

Preparation Time: 15 minutes
Cooking Time: 25 minutes
Servings: 4
Ingredients :
- 4 Portobello mushroom caps

- 1 tablespoon olive oil

- 1/2 teaspoon salt, divided

- ¼ teaspoon freshly ground black pepper, divided

- 1 cup baby spinach, chopped

- 11/2 cups part-skim ricotta cheese

- 1/2 cup part-skim shredded mozzarella cheese

- ¼ cup grated parmesan cheese

- 1 garlic clove, minced

- 1 tablespoon dried parsley

- 2 teaspoons dried oregano

- 4 teaspoons unseasoned bread crumbs, divided

- 4 servings (4 cups) roasted broccoli with shallots

Directions:
1. Preheat the oven to 375f. Line a baking sheet with aluminum foil.

2. Brush the mushroom caps with the olive oil, and sprinkle with ¼ teaspoon salt and 1/8 teaspoon pepper. Put the mushroom caps on the prepared baking sheet and bake until soft, about 12 minutes.

3. In a medium bowl, mix together the spinach, ricotta, mozzarella, parmesan, garlic, parsley, oregano, and the remaining ¼ teaspoon of salt and 1/8 teaspoon of pepper.

4. Spoon 1/2 cup of cheese mixture into each mushroom cap, and sprinkle each with 1 teaspoon of bread crumbs. Return the mushrooms to the oven for an additional 8 to 10 minutes until warmed through.

5. Remove from the oven and allow the mushrooms to cool for about 10 minutes before placing each in an individual container. Add 1 cup of roasted broccoli with shallots to each container.

Nutrition:
calories: 419;

total fat: 30g;

saturated fat: 10g;

protein: 23g;

total carbs: 19g;

fiber: 2g;

sugar: 3g;

sodium: 790mg

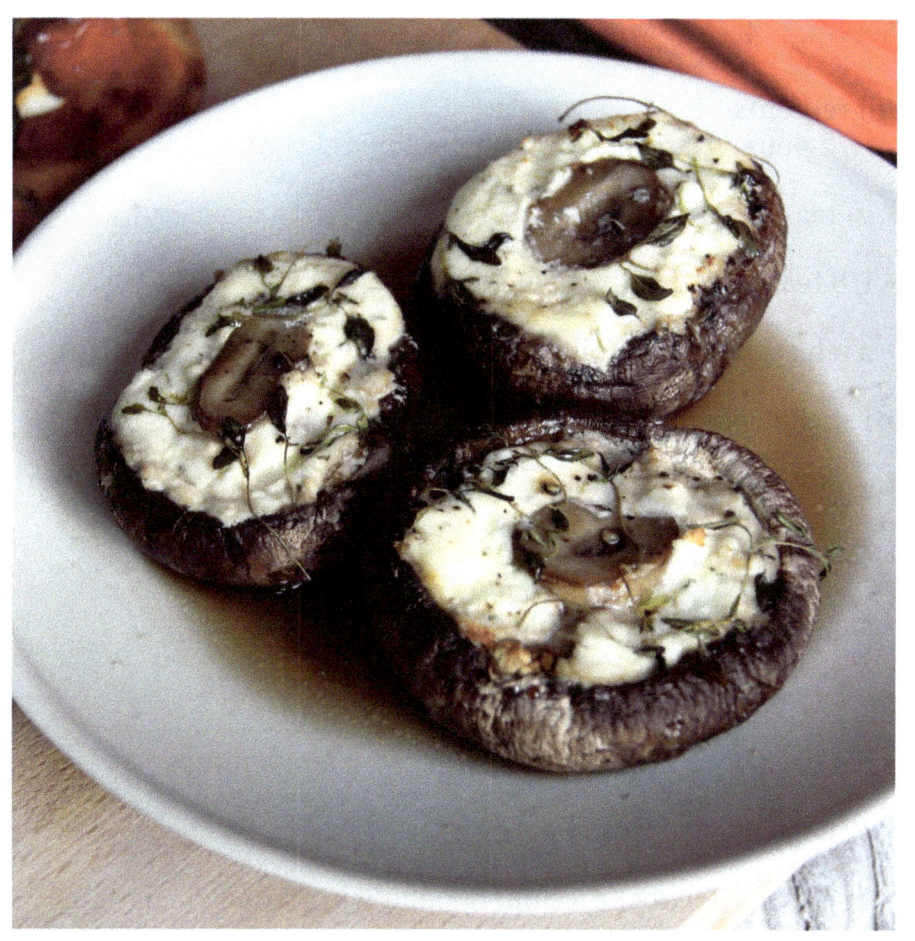

Lighter Shrimp Scampi

Preparation Time: 15 minutes
Cooking Time: 15 minutes
Servings: 4

Ingredients :
- 11/2 pounds large peeled and deveined shrimp

- ¼ teaspoon salt

- 1/8 teaspoon freshly ground black pepper

- 2 tablespoons olive oil

- 1 shallot, chopped

- 2 garlic cloves, minced

- ¼ cup cooking white wine

- Juice of 1/2 lemon (1 tablespoon)

- 1/2 teaspoon sriracha

- 2 tablespoons unsalted butter, at room temperature

- ¼ cup chopped fresh parsley

- 4 servings (6 cups) zucchini noodles with lemon vinaigrette

Directions:
1. Season the shrimp with the salt and pepper.

2. In a medium saucepan over medium heat, heat the oil. Add the shallot and garlic, and cook until the shallot softens and the garlic is fragrant, about 3 minutes. Add the shrimp, cover, and cook until opaque, 2 to 3 minutes on each side. Using a slotted spoon, transfer the shrimp to a large plate.

3. Add the wine, lemon juice, and sriracha to the saucepan, and stir to combine. Bring the mixture to a boil, then reduce the heat and simmer until the liquid is reduced by about half, 3 minutes. Add the butter and stir until melted, about 3 minutes. Return the shrimp to the saucepan and toss to coat. Add the parsley and stir to combine.

4. Into each of 4 containers, place 11/2 cups of zucchini noodles with lemon vinaigrette, and top with ¾ cup of scampi.

Nutrition:
calories: 364;

total fat: 21g;

saturated fat: 6g;

protein: 37g;

total carbs: 10g;

fiber: 2g;

sugar: 6g;

sodium: 557mg

Maple-Mustard Salmon

Preparation Time: 10 minutes, plus 30 minutes marinating time

Cooking Time: 20 minutes
Servings: 4

Ingredients :
- Nonstick cooking spray

- 1/2 cup 100% maple syrup

- 2 tablespoons Dijon mustard

- ¼ teaspoon salt

- 4 (5-ounce) salmon fillets

- 4 servings (4 cups) roasted broccoli with shallots

- 4 servings (2 cups) parsleyed whole-wheat couscous

Directions:
1. Preheat the oven to 400f. Line a baking sheet with aluminum foil and coat with cooking spray.

2. In a medium bowl, whisk together the maple syrup, mustard, and salt until smooth.

3. Put the salmon fillets into the bowl and toss to coat. Cover and place in the refrigerator to marinate for at least 30 minutes and up to overnight.

4. Shake off excess marinade from the salmon fillets and place them on the prepared baking sheet, leaving a 1-inch space between each fillet. Discard the extra marinade.

5. Bake for about 20 minutes until the salmon is opaque and a thermometer inserted in the thickest part of a fillet reads 145f.

6. Into each of 4 resealable containers, place 1 salmon fillet, 1 cup of roasted broccoli with shallots, and 1/2 cup of parsleyed whole-wheat couscous.

Nutrition:
calories: 601;

total fat: 29g;

saturated fat: 4g;

protein: 36g;

total carbs: 51g;

fiber: 3g;

sugar: 23g;

sodium: 610mg

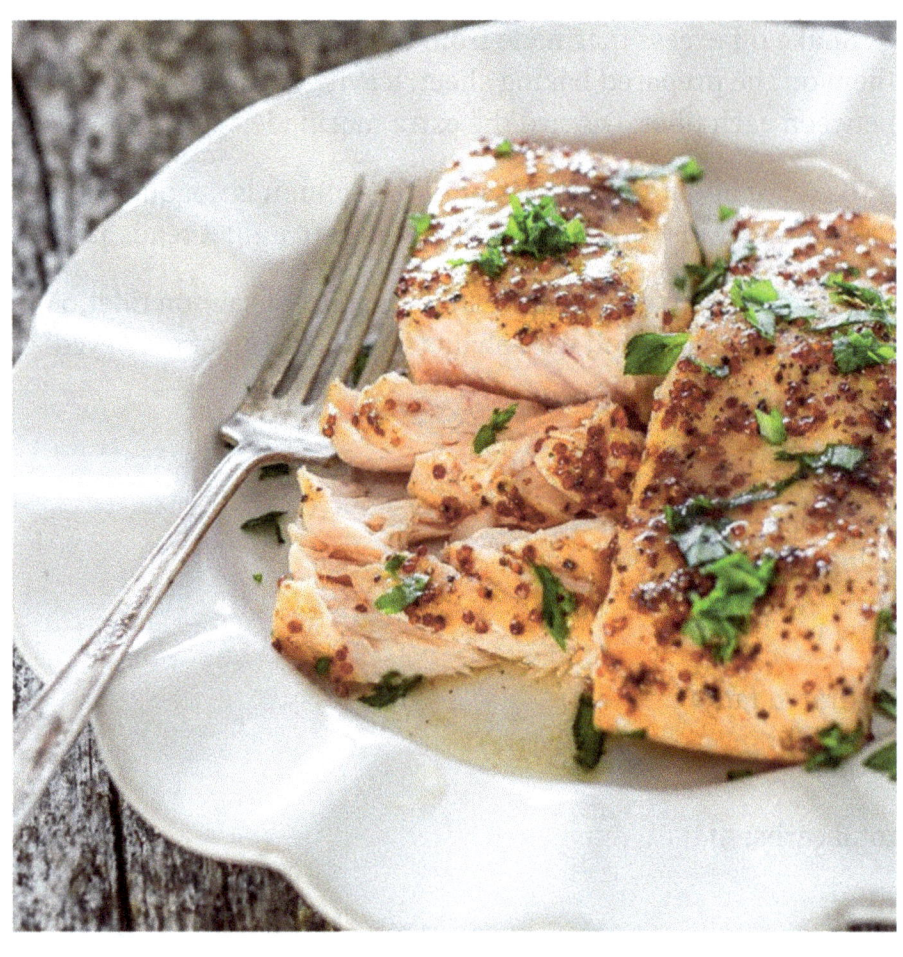

Chicken Salad With Grapes And Pecans

Preparation Time: 15 Minutes
Cooking Time: 5 Minutes
Servings: 4

Ingredients :

- 1/3 cup unsalted pecans, chopped

- 10 ounces cooked skinless, boneless chicken breast or rotisserie chicken, finely chopped

- 1/2 medium yellow onion, finely chopped

- 1 celery stalk, finely chopped

- ¾ cup red or green seedless grapes, halved

- ¼ cup light mayonnaise

- ¼ cup nonfat plain Greek yogurt

- 1 tablespoon Dijon mustard

- 1 tablespoon dried parsley

- ¼ teaspoon salt

- 1/8 teaspoon freshly ground black pepper

- 1 cup shredded romaine lettuce

- 4 (8-inch) whole-wheat pitas

Directions:
1. Heat a small skillet over medium-low heat to toast the pecans. Cook the pecans until fragrant, about 3 minutes. Remove from the heat and set aside to cool.

2. In a medium bowl, mix the chicken, onion, celery, pecans, and grapes.

3. In a small bowl, whisk together the mayonnaise, yogurt, mustard, parsley, salt, and pepper. Spoon the sauce over the chicken mixture and stir until well combined.

4. Into each of 4 containers, place ¼ cup of lettuce and top with 1 cup of chicken salad. Store the pitas separately until ready to serve.

5. When ready to eat, stuff the serving of salad and lettuce into 1 pita.

Nutrition:
Calories: 418;

Total Fat: 14g;

Saturated Fat: 2g;

Protein: 31g;

Total Carbs: 43g;

Fiber: 6g;

Courgettes In Cider Sauce

Preparation Time: 13 minutes
Cooking Time: 17 minutes
Servings: 3

Ingredients :
- 2 cups baby courgettes

- 3 tablespoons vegetable stock

- 2 tablespoons apple cider vinegar

- 1 tablespoon light brown sugar

- 4 spring onions, finely sliced

- 1 piece fresh gingerroot, grated

- 1 teaspoon corn flour

- 2 teaspoons water

Directions:
1. Bring a pan with salted water to a boil. Add courgettes. Bring to a boil for 5 minutes.

2. Meanwhile, in a pan, combine vegetable stock, apple cider vinegar, brown sugar, onions, gingerroot, lemon juice and rind, and orange juice and rind. Take to a boil. Lower the heat and allow simmering for 3 minutes.

3. Mix the corn flour with water. Stir well. Pour into the sauce. Continue stirring until the sauce thickens.

4. Drain courgettes. Transfer to the serving dish. Spoon over the sauce. Toss to coat courgettes. Serve.

Nutrition:
Calories 173

Total Fat 9. 2 g

Saturated Fat 0.8 g

Cholesterol 0 mg

Sodium 861 mg

Total Carbs 22. 5 g

Fiber 6. 3 g

Sugar 2. 3 g

Protein 9. 2 g

Baked Mixed Mushrooms

Preparation Time: 8 minutes
Cooking Time: 20 minutes
Servings: 3

Ingredients :
- 2 cups mixed wild mushrooms
- 1 cup chestnut mushrooms
- 2 cups dried porcini
- 2 shallots
- 4 garlic cloves
- 3 cups raw pecans
- ½ bunch fresh thyme
- 1 bunch flat-leaf parsley
- 2 tablespoons olive oil
- 2 fresh bay leaves
- 1 ½ cups stale bread

Directions:
1. Remove skin and finely chop garlic and shallots. Roughly chop the wild mushrooms and chestnut mushrooms. Pick the leaves of the thyme and tear the bread into small pieces. Put inside the pressure cooker.

2. Place the pecans and roughly chop the nuts. Pick the parsley leaves and roughly chop.

3. Place the porcini in a bowl then add 300ml of boiling water. Set aside until needed.

4. Heat oil in the pressure cooker. Add the garlic and shallots. Cook for 3 minutes while stirring occasionally.

5. Drain porcini and reserve the liquid. Add the porcini into the pressure cooker together with the wild mushrooms and chestnut mushrooms. Add the bay leaves and thyme.

6. Position the lid and lock in place. Put to high heat and bring to high pressure. Adjust heat to stabilize. Cook for 10 minutes. Adjust taste if necessary.

7. Transfer the mushroom mixture into a bowl and set aside to cool completely.

8. Once the mushrooms are completely cool, add the bread, pecans, a pinch of black pepper and sea salt, and half of the reserved liquid into the bowl. Mix well. Add more reserved liquid if the mixture seems dry.

9. Add more than half of the parsley into the bowl and stir. Transfer the mixture into a 20cm x 25cm lightly greased baking dish and cover with tin foil.

10. Bake in the oven for 35 minutes. Then, get rid of the foil and cook for another 10 minutes. Once done, sprinkle the remaining parsley on top and serve with bread or crackers. Serve.

Nutrition:
Calories 343

Total Fat 4. 2 g

Saturated Fat 0.8 g

Cholesterol 0 mg

Sodium 861 mg

Total Carbs 22. 5 g

Fiber 6. 3 g

Sugar 2. 3 g

Protein 9. 2 g

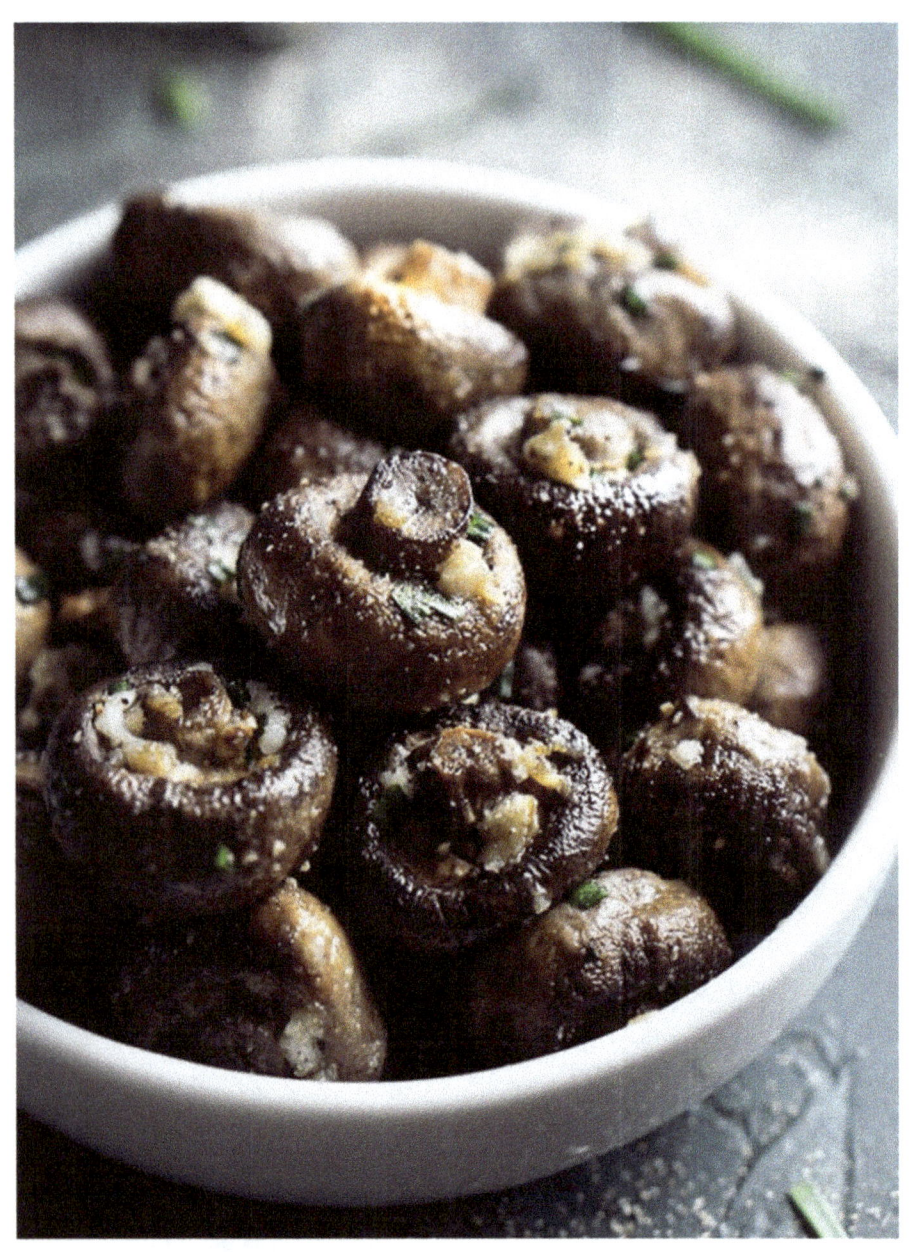

Spiced Okra

Preparation Time: 14 minutes
Cooking Time: 16 minutes
Servings: 3

Ingredients :
- 2 cups okra

- ¼ teaspoon stevia

- 1 teaspoon chilli powder

- ½ teaspoon ground turmeric

- 1 tablespoon ground coriander

- 2 tablespoons fresh coriander, chopped

- 1 tablespoon ground cumin

- ¼ teaspoon salt

- 1 tablespoon desiccated coconut

- 3 tablespoons vegetable oil

- ½ teaspoon black mustard seeds

- ½ teaspoon cumin seeds

- Fresh tomatoes, to garnish

Directions:
1. Trim okra. Wash and dry.

2. Combine stevia, chilli powder, turmeric, ground coriander, fresh coriander, cumin, salt, and desiccated coconut in a bowl.

3. Heat the oil in a pan. Cook mustard and cumin seeds for 3 minutes. Stir continuously. Add okra. Tip in the spice mixture. Cook on low heat for 8 minutes.

4. Transfer to a serving dish. Garnish with fresh tomatoes.

Nutrition:
Calories 163

Total Fat 4. 2 g

Saturated Fat 0.8 g

Cholesterol 0 mg

Sodium 861 mg

Total Carbs 22. 5 g

Fiber 6. 3 g

Sugar 2. 3 g

Protein 9. 2 g

Alkalizing Green Soup

Preparation Time: 10 Minutes
Cooking Time: 10 minutes
Servings: 2

Ingredients
- 1 tablespoon sunflower or coconut oil
- 1 pint of stock made with 1 tablespoon vegetable Bouillon powder
- 1/4 tablespoon fennel seeds
- ½ red onion- finely chopped
- 1 cup tender stem broccoli
- 1¼ cups baby spinach
- Juice and zest of 1 lemon
- 1 clove garlic- finely chopped

Directions:
1. Fry the garlic, red onions, and fennel seeds in oil over medium heat for about 2 minutes.

2. Add in the broccoli, zest, stock and lemon juice and let it cook for 4 minutes.

3. Remove from heat and toss in the baby spinach. Stir until the spinach is wilted.

4. Immediately add the mixture to a blender and blend until smooth.

Nutrition:
Calories: 218

Healing Ginger Carrot Soup

Preparation Time: 10 Minutes
Cooking Time: 15 minutes
Servings: 2

Ingredients
- 1 tablespoon fresh ginger

- Sea salt and pepper- to taste

- 2 garlic cloves

- ½ onion- quartered

- 4 carrots- washed and peeled

- 2 cups vegetable stock

- 1 teaspoon turmeric

Directions:
1. Add all your **Ingredients** to a large pot and bring to a boil. Once boiled, let it simmer for 30 minutes. When the carrots are soft, blend using an immersion blender until smooth.

2. Garnish with some hemp seeds on top if desired.

3. Enjoy!

Nutrition:
Calories: 210

Kale Salad

Preparation Time: 10 Minutes
Cooking Time: 0 minutes
Servings: 2

Ingredients
Salad

- ½ (or a whole) avocado

- 2 handfuls of sprouts (any kind)

- 1 head lacinato kale (also called dinosaur kale)

- 1 medium-to large tomato

Dressing

- ½ tablespoon olive oil (optional)

- 1 teaspoon Dijon mustard

- 4 drops liquid stevia

- 4 Tablespoons Nutritional yeast

- Juice of 1 lemon

- Cayenne pepper to taste

Optional toppings:

- Sunflower or pumpkin seeds

- A few strips of seared tempeh

- Regular tempeh

Directions:
1. Discard the kale stems (can discard or keep for juicing later on) and use your hands to tear up the kale into bite sized pieces. Put the kale in a large bowl.

2. Sprinkle some salt and massage for a couple of minutes to help break down the kale.

3. Combine the dressing Ingredients in a small bowl. Mix it into the kale by massaging (don't be afraid to get your hands dirty as this will help make the kale softer).

4. Cut the toppings and add to the salad bowl.

5. Toss and serve right away.

Nutrition:
Calories: 248

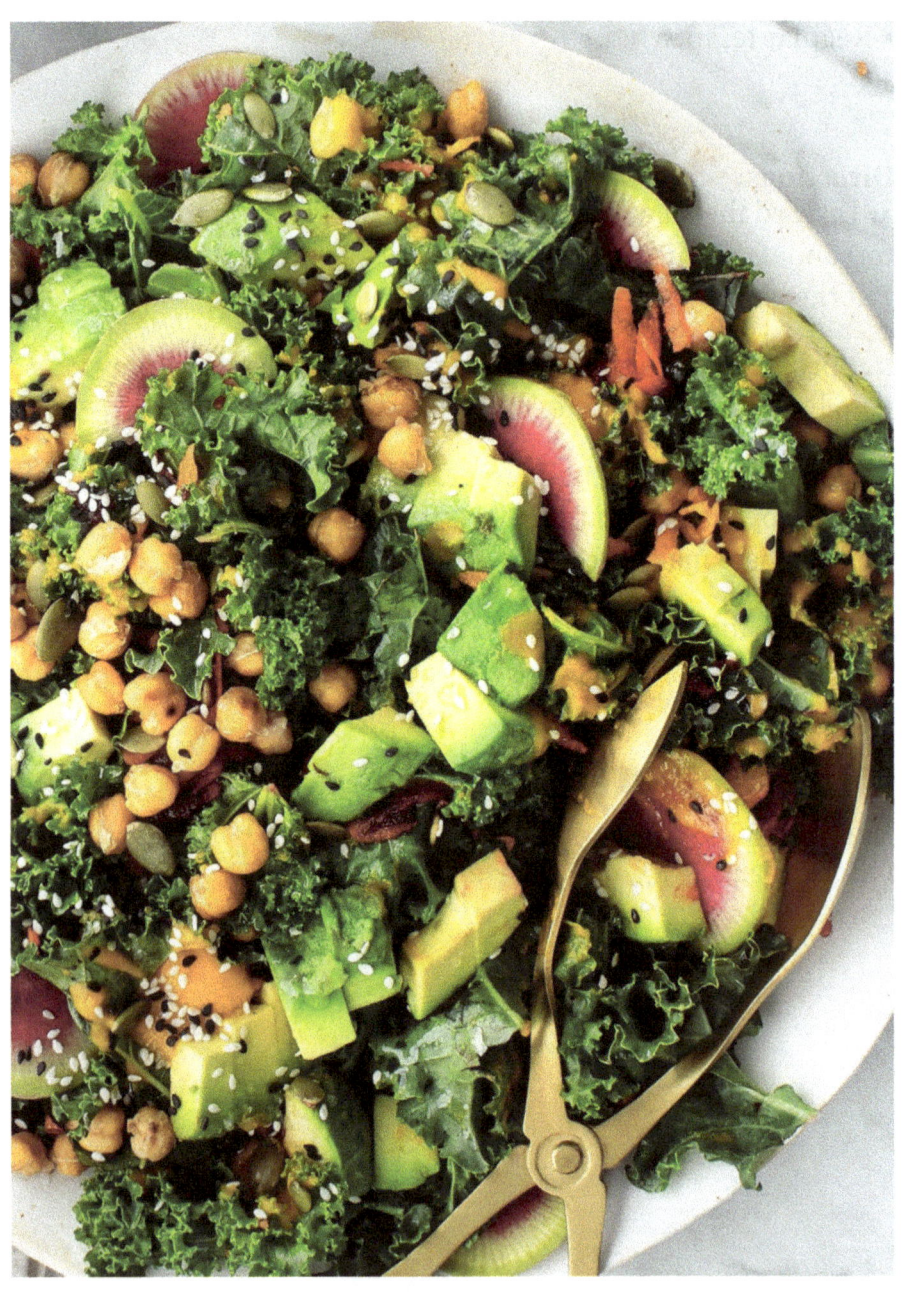

Turmeric Curry And Roasted Cauliflower

Preparation Time: 10 Minutes
Cooking Time: 35 minutes

Servings: 4

Before I commence, it is worthy to note that four of the most potent anti-inflammatory foods are represented in this meal i.e., bell pepper, turmeric, ginger, and garlic.

On the other hand, the coconut oil, seeds, and nuts present in this meal are also sources of healthy fats. So, when you eat this meal, be assured that you are doing a big favor to your body's immune system

This delicious meal is alkaline, anti-inflammatory and also possesses healthy fats. Copy this recipe today and get in the groove.

Ingredients :
Ingredients for the CURRY

- Turmeric powder, one (1) teaspoon

- Water, 1 ½ cups

- Himalayan salt, 1 teaspoon

- Garam masala, ½ teaspoon

- Chili powder, ½ teaspoon

- Red onions (finely chopped), 2 cups

- Cauliflowers (floret), 2 cups
- Salt, ½ teaspoon
- Roma tomatoes (finely chopped), ½ cup
- Bell pepper/capsicum (diced), 1
- Coriander (chopped), 1 tablespoon
- Coconut milk (unsweetened), 2 cups
- Coconut oil, 2 tablespoons
- Garlic (minced), 3 cloves
- Ginger powder, 1 teaspoon
- Turmeric (fresh), 1cm

Ingredients for Masala

- Cloves, 6
- Cumin seeds, 1 tablespoon
- Coriander seeds, 1 ½ tablespoons
- Cinnamon stick, 1 ¼ inch
- Raw cashew, ½ cup
- Cardamom powder, 1 pinch

Directions:
1. First of all, preheat the oven to 200°C

2. Get a large mixing bowl and add the powdered turmeric, coconut oil, a pinch of salt and the cauliflower.

3. Use your hands and mix them together properly.

4. Now, get a baking tray lined with baking powder and pour the mix into it.

5. Put it in the oven for twenty to thirty minutes.

6. Mind you, do not let the cauliflower burn.

7. While the cauliflower is cooking in the oven, we shift our attention to the Masala.

8. To make the Masala, blend all the masala Ingredients in a food processor and make sure it is completely smooth.

9. Next, get a large pan and heat the coconut oil over a gentle heat.

10. Add garlic, ginger, and onions and cook gently between two to three minutes.

11. Next, add bell pepper/capsicum and tomatoes.

12. Cook until tomatoes begin to fall apart.

13. Now add the masala mix and stir for two to three minutes.

14. Keep stirring to avoid it from sticking or getting burnt.

15. Once its thoroughly mixed, add chili pepper, turmeric, and coconut milk, as well as, water (as much as you desire).

16. Reduce the heat down to simmer and allow it to cook for five minutes.

17. Season to taste.

18. When cauliflower is done, take it away from the oven and add to the pan.

19. Mix it thoroughly.

20. Switch of the heat.

22. When you decide to serve, stir through the cilantro/coriander.

22. Serve!

23. You can have it with brown rice or quinoa.

Nutrition:
Calories: 163

Alkaline Tortilla Soup

Preparation Time: 15 Minutes
Cooking Time: 10 minutes

Servings: 4

Tortilla soup is a good-looking blend of healthy and alkalized food Ingredients entwined together to make a tasty and spicy meal.

It is rich in flavor, nutrients such as calcium, potassium, vitamins A, B and K, manganese, magnesium, and copper. This meal contains properties that help reduce blood cholesterol, fight cancer and cleanse the colon.

The taste of this meal is super!

Ingredients :
- Tomato, one (1)

- Lime, one (1)

- Avocado (ripe), one (1)

- Water (filtered), 500ml

- Coriander (cilantro), ½ bunch

- Garlic, two (2) cloves

- Red Capsicum (pepper), ½

- Spinach, two (2) large handfuls

- Vegetable bouillon, two (2) teaspoons

- Corn (on the cob), one (1)
- Sprouted tortilla wrap, one (1)
- Cayenne pepper, (a pinch)
- Himalayan salt and black pepper, (a pinch)
- Jalapeno/chili, one (1)

Directions:
1. Slice your tortilla into 5cm long and 1cm wide strips and toast lightly under a grill

2. Next, get a large pan and add water.

3. Boil over medium heat and dissolve the bouillon/stock cubes.

4. The idea is to make a vegetable broth as the base.

5. Time to prepare the veggies; chop the coriander roughly and dice the tomato and capsicum.

6. Finely mince the garlic, peel and dice the avocado.

7. Slice your chili or jalapeno depending on your preference and set on one side.

8. Wash and chop the spinach and move on to the corn.

9. To prepare the corn, use a sharp knife to slice off the kernels from the cob.

10. Next, throw everything in the broth and heat.

11. Turn off the heat in a few minutes.

12. Food is ready.

Nutrition:
Calories: 157

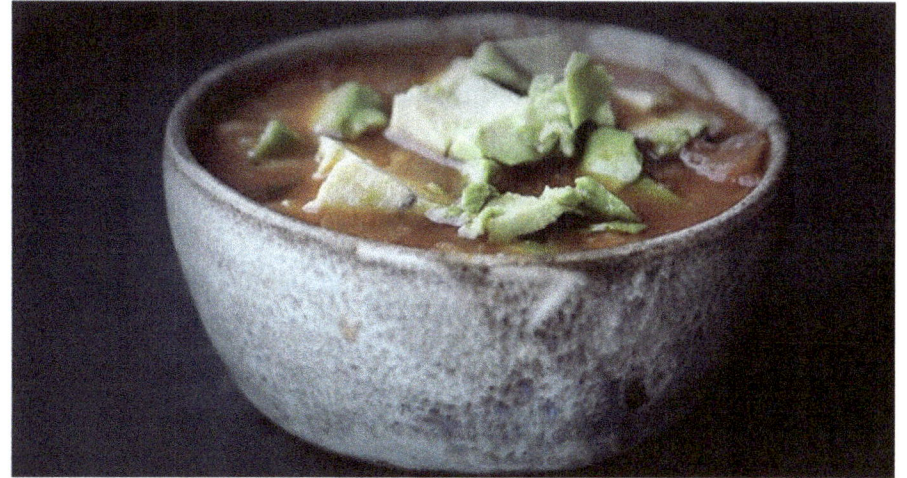

Hearty Minestrone

Preparation Time: 15 Minutes
Cooking Time: 15 minutes
Servings: 2

The hearty Minestrone is loaded with alkaline and fantastically tasty at the same time. So when you settle for it, you are only doing your body a huge favor. Aubergine is rich in minerals, manganese, fiber and a host of other vitamins, as well as phytonutrients, which are antioxidants.

When you consider the combination of carrot, zucchini, and sweet potato in this meal, you'll be left with no doubt that the Hearty Minestrone is delicious, nutritious, and healthy.

Ingredients :
- Basil, one (1) handful

- Carrot, ½ cup

- Sweet potato, ½ cup

- Red onion, ¼

- Coconut oil, one (1) tablespoon

- Aubergine (eggplant), ½ cup

- Vegetable stock, one (1) cup

- Zucchini (courgette), ½ cup

- Tomato juice (fresh/bought), 1 cup

- Beans, ½ cup

- Carrot, ½ cup

- Black pepper and Himalayan salt

Directions:
1. Wash and dice the onion and carrot.

2. Cube the courgette, aubergine, and potato.

3. Next fry the onion, carrot, courgette, aubergine, and potato in a large pot for two minutes.

4. Add the tomato juice, the stock, and beans.

5. Bring it to a boil and reduce the heat to simmer for eight to ten minutes.

6. Add the basil and stir.

7. Season to taste.

Nutrition:
Calories: 110

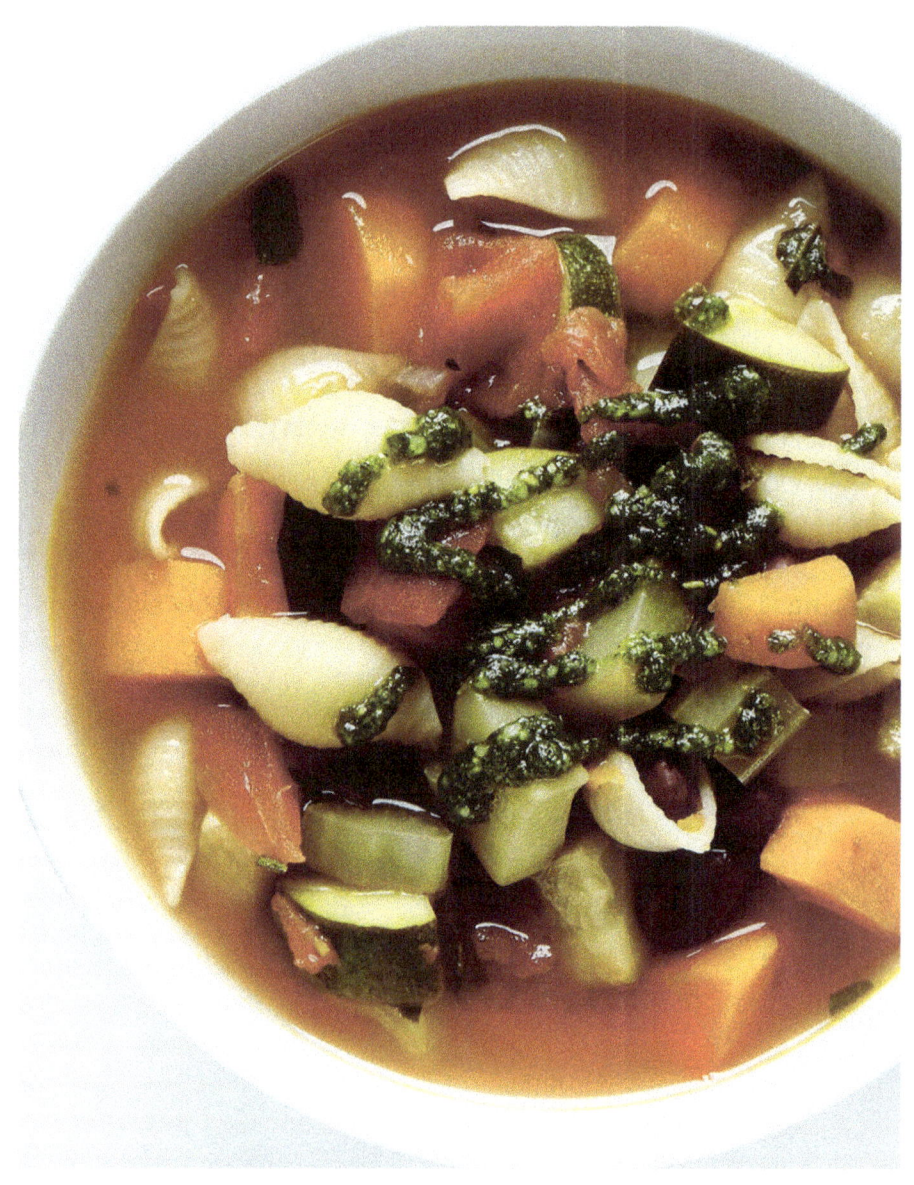

Raw Pad Thai (With Zucchini Noodles)

Preparation Time: 15 Minutes
Cooking Time: 10 minutes
Servings: 2

This simple recipe is raw, nutrient-rich and tastes extremely good. The fact that it is readily accepted by even non-alkalizer is a testament of how good it tastes. I had put this recipe to the test by serving it at one of our hiking club end of year parties and to my greatest surprise; it was well received by everyone that had it. A lot of people came to me directly, asking what this strange meal was and how they could go about preparing it.

It is a delightful meal and I urge you to take some time out to explore it and thank me later.

Ingredients :
- Carrots (large), three (3)

- Cauliflower (floret), one (1)

- Beansprouts, ½ packet

- Red cabbage (shredded), one (1) cup

- Courgettes (Zucchini), three (3) medium sizes

- Spring onions (chopped)

- Coconut oil

- Coriander/cilantro (fresh and roughly chopped), one (1) bunch

Ingredients for Sauce

- Ginger root (grated), one (1) inch
- Tahini, ¼ cup
- Tamari, ¼ cup
- Lemon/lime juice, two (2) teaspoon
- Almond butter, ¼ cup
- Garlic (minced), one (1) clove
- Coconut sugar, one (1) teaspoon

Directions:
1. Start with the courgette and carrot noodles: use a mandolin or vegetable peeler to slice both and then use a knife to slice them into thin strips.

2. Get a large bowl and add them, alongside the shredded cabbage, coriander, spring onions, cauliflower, and beansprouts.

3. For the sauce; blend the grated ginger, tahini, garlic, lime/lemon juice, tamari, almond butter, and coconut sugar.

4. Add some water and blast till a thick sauce is formed.

5. Finally, get a bowl and mix the sauce inside.

6. Serve with a little squeeze of lime/lemon and a spring of coriander.

Nutrition:
Calories: 229

Spinach Quinoa

Preparation Time: 10 minutes.
Cooking Time: 25 minutes.

Servings: 4
Ingredients :
- 1 cup quinoa

- 2 cups fresh spinach, chopped

- 1 ½ cups filtered alkaline water

- 1 sweet potato, peeled and cubed

- 1 tsp. coriander powder

- 1 tsp. turmeric

- 1 tsp. cumin seeds

- 1 tsp. fresh ginger, grated

- 2 garlic cloves, chopped

- 1 cup onion, chopped

- 2 tbsp. olive oil

- 1 fresh lime juice

- Pepper

- Salt

Directions:
1. Add oil in the instant pot and set the pot on sauté mode.

2. Add the onion in olive oil and sauté for 2 minutes or until onion is softened.

3. Add garlic, ginger, spices, and quinoa and cook for 3–4 minutes.

4. Add spinach, sweet potatoes, and water and stir well.

5. Seal pot with lid and cook on manual high pressure for 2 minutes.

6. When finished, allow releasing pressure naturally then open the lid.

7. Add lime juice and stir well.

8. Serve and enjoy.

Nutrition:
Calories: 268

Fat: 9. 9 g.

Carbohydrates: 38. 8 g.

Sugar: 3. 4 g.

Protein: 7. 6 g.

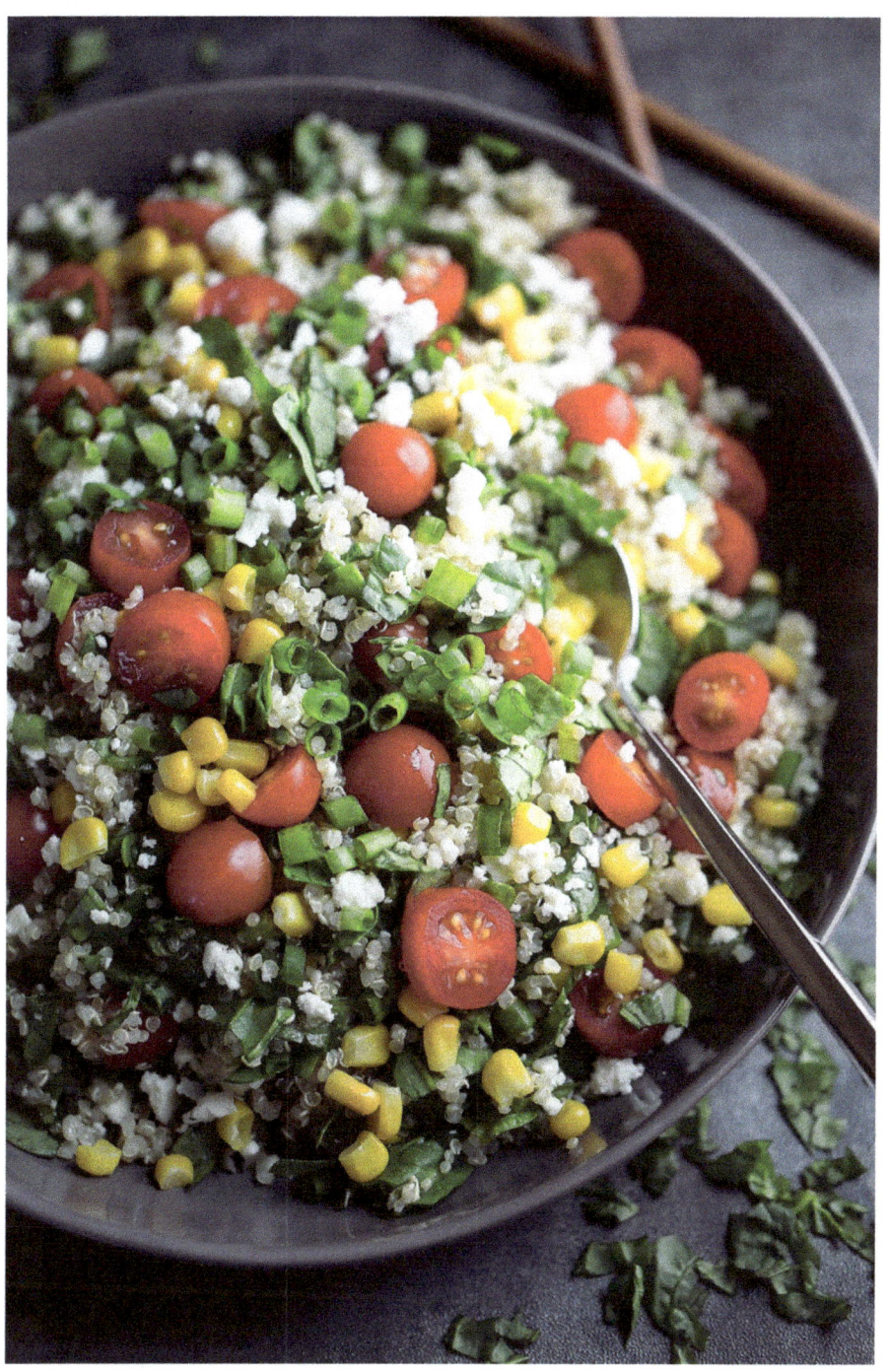

Spicy Eggplant

Preparation Time: 15 minutes.
Cooking Time: 5 minutes.
Servings: 4

Ingredients :
- 1 eggplant, cut into 1–inch cubes
- ½ cup filtered alkaline water
- 1 cup tomato, chopped
- ½ tsp. Italian seasoning
- 1 tsp. paprika
- ½ tsp. red pepper
- 1 tsp. garlic powder
- 2 tbsp. extra virgin olive oil
- ¼ tsp. sea salt

Directions:
1. Add eggplant and water into the instant pot.

2. Seal pot with lid and cook on manual high pressure for 5 minutes.

3. When finished, release pressure using the quick-release method than open the lid. Drain eggplant well.

4. Add oil in an instant pot and set a pot on sauté mode.

5. Return eggplant in the pot along with tomato, Italian seasoning, paprika, red pepper, garlic powder, and salt and stir until combined.

6. Cook on sauté mode for 5 minutes. Stir occasionally.

7. Serve and enjoy.

Nutrition:
Calories: 107

Fat: 7. 6 g.

Carbohydrates: 10.5 g.

Sugar: 5. 6 g.

Protein: 1. 9 g.

Cholesterol: 0 mg.

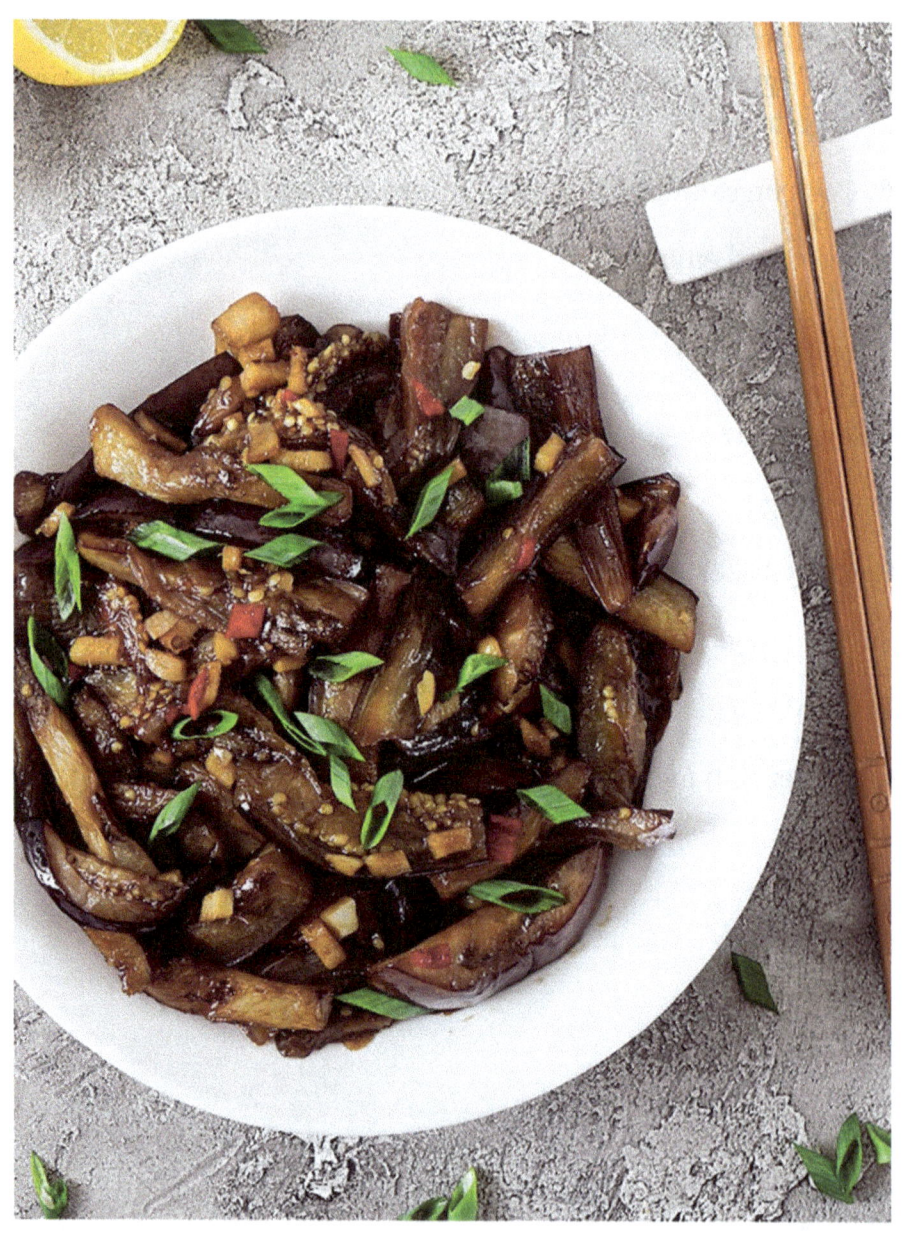

www.ingramcontent.com/pod-product-compliance
Lightning Source LLC
Chambersburg PA
CBHW070725030426
42336CB00013B/1917